The Lectin Free Cookbook

Healthy Recipes for Your Electric Pressure Cooker

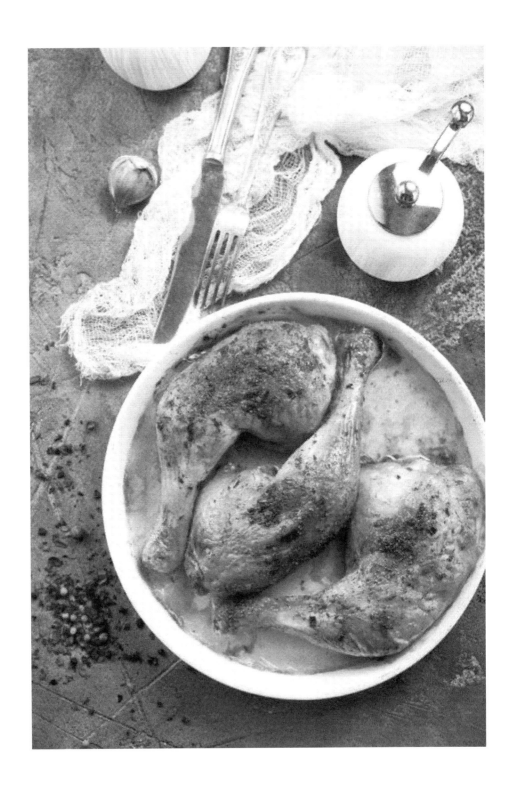

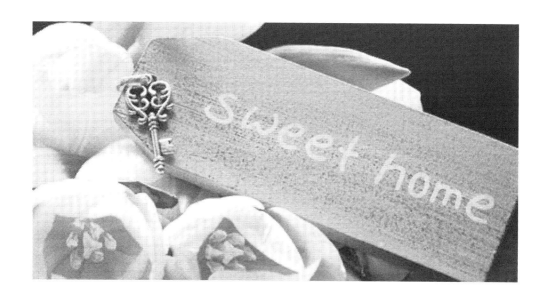

Please, leave your review of the book, if you have a free minute. Your feedback is essential for other readers and for us to make the right choice.

Table of Contents

TABLE OF CONTENTS 4

INTRODUCTION 7

BASICS OF THE LECTIN FREE DIET 9

    WHAT ARE LECTINS? 9

    HOW LECTINS CAN HARM YOUR HEALTH? 10

    WHAT IS A LECTIN FREE DIET? 11

    BENEFITS OF A LECTIN FREE DIET 13

    LECTIN-FREE PANTRY STAPLES AND SEASONINGS 14

    WHAT IS AN INSTANT POT? 17

    ADVANTAGES OF INSTANT POT 18

SOUPS 20

    CHICKEN KALE SOUP 20

    CHICKEN TURMERIC SOUP 22

    THAI BROCCOLI AND BEEF SOUP 25

    ROASTED GARLIC SOUP 27

    HAMBURGER VEGETABLE SOUP 29

VEGETABLE RECIPES 31

    SESAME BOK CHOY PLATTER 31

    COOL INSTANT POT BROCCOLI 33

    AWESOME PARSNIPS AND CHIVE SOUP 35

    SUBTLE BRAISED CABBAGE 37

    DELICIOUS BOWL OF MUSHROOMS 39

    YUMMY ROASTED ARTICHOKE PLATTER 41

    FEISTY POT OF BRUSSELS SPROUTS 43

    CREAMY LEEK AND BROCCOLI SOUP 45

    GARLIC AND BROCCOLI MASH 47

    HEALTHY CARROT SOUP 49

SEAFOOD RECIPES 51

- Fantastic Ginger Tilapia 51
- Pepper Lemon Salmon 54
- Gentle Crab Legs 56
- Slightly Spicy Chili Salmon 58
- Juicy Coconut Fish Curry 60

PORK RECIPES 62

- Hearty Lemon and Artichoke Pork Chops 62
- Tender Soft Pineapple Pork Chops 64
- Onion Pork Bliss 66
- Easy Jamaican Pork 68
- Sprouts and Chops Medley 70
- Shredded Cabbage and Bacon 72
- The "Ghee"- Licious Pork Chops 73
- Olive Dredged Pork Belly 75

BEEF RECIPES 77

- Exotic Chili and Garlic Beef 77
- Broccoli and Ginger Beef 79
- Spicy Tourne Beef 81
- Balsamic Beef Delight 83
- Rich Beef Stew 85
- South Beef Stir Fry 87
- Original Texas Beef Chili 89

POULTRY RECIPES 91

- Feisty Turkey Wings 91
- Amazing Chicken Primavera 93
- Caramelized Onion Chicken 95
- Simple and Precious Chinese Chicken 97
- The Healthy "FAUX" Chicken Taco 98
- All-Time Favorite Orange Chicken 99
- Delicious Lemon Chicken and Cauliflower Mash 101

SALAD RECIPES 103

- AWESOME CITRUS AND CAULIFLOWER SALAD 103
- EXTREMELY HEARTY BEET SALAD 105
- CAPER AND BEET SALAD 107
- CRAZY CARROT AND KALE MEDLEY 109

DESSERTS RECIPES 111

- COOL PEPPERMINT LATTE 111
- VERY CREAMY MASHED SWEET POTATOES 113
- PEACHY RASPBERRY LEMONADE 115
- HEARTY COCONUT AND AVOCADO PUDDING 117
- EASY BAKED APPLE 119
- CREATIVE STINKING ROSE 121
- HEARTY SWEET AND SPICY CARROT 123

COOKING MEASUREMENT CONVERSION 125

GROCERY SHOPPING LIST 126

OUR RECOMMENDATIONS 129

ABOUT THE AUTHOR 130

RECIPE INDEX 131

Introduction

So, what are lectins, and why do people avoid this food substance?

Certain foods—like grain, beans, fruits, vegetables, and conventional dairy products—contain amounts of protein compounds called **lectins** that are found to be highly toxic. Effects of these protein compounds include inflammation in the body, brain fog, an increase in weight, and other digestive issues.

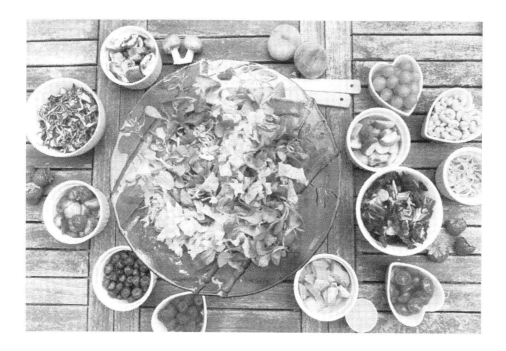

- ***A lectin-free diet is a deduction diet to eliminate food products that have high amounts of lectins for people who are highly sensitive to these protein substances.***

In this day and age, people are caught in the trend of being busy and distracted. People are mostly unaware of what is happening to their bodies, which sometimes is manifested by feeling tired, bloated, or heavy. Then year after year, weight continues to add on.

By being aware of the possible outcomes when foods containing lectin are avoided in the diet, it can be an excellent reward for the changes to the body when it is being filled only with nourishing and real food.

One of the challenges that may arise in starting this diet could be the time needed to prepare these meals. Having that in mind, this recipe book is focused on using one of the most sought-after tools in the kitchen—the instant pot.

This kitchen tool is a combination of an electric pressure cooker, rice cooker, even yogurt maker and slow cooker. And rest assured that even beginners can manage to use it.

Basics of the Lectin Free Diet

What are Lectins?

Lectins are a type of protein that binds to carbohydrates in the digestive tract. They are **macromolecules** that are highly specific for **sugar moieties** of other molecules. Lectins make **molecules stick together without influencing the immune system**, which can **affect cell-cell interaction**. Lectins also mediate the attachment and binding of bacteria and viruses to their intended targets.

Lectins are abundant in

- **nightshade vegetables, such as tomatoes, potatoes, goji berries, peppers, and eggplant**
- **all legumes, such as lentils, beans, chickpeas, and peanuts**
- **peanut-based products, such as peanut butter and peanut oil**
- **all grains and products made with grain or flour, including cakes, crackers, and bread**
- **dairy products, such as milk**

How Lectins Can Harm Your Health?

- **Autoimmune diseases**

  Lectin penetrates into the gut wall causing a robust immune response due to its negative autoimmune and inflammatory effects.

- **Anti-nutrients**

  Lectin reduces absorption and digestion of food in the gut thus acting as an "antinutrient." This means they have a detrimental effect on your gut microbiome by shifting the balance of your bacterial flora.

- **Weight gain**

  Lectin has been said to be a significant culprit in unexplained weight gain in humans.

- **Rheumatoid Arthritis**

  Lectins act as proteins in the thyroid and joints thereby attacking the thyroid gland and contributing to rheumatoid arthritis.

> **Bloating**

Consuming lectins in large amounts results in gastric distress in most people.

What is a Lectin Free Diet?

A lectin-free diet is simply a reduction in the intake of high-lectin foods or the complete elimination of lectin from one's daily diet.

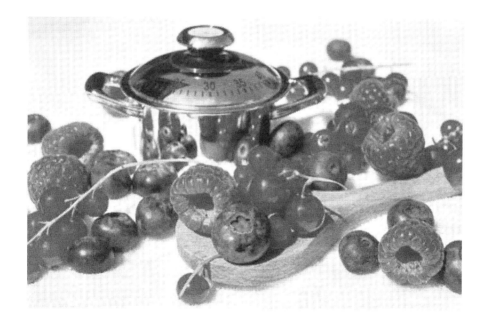

Examples of lectin-free foods you can start eating now are:

- **Fruits and Vegetables:** romaine lettuce, oranges, lemons, cruciferous vegetables, cherries, cucumbers, celery, onion, broccoli, cauliflower, mushrooms, pumpkin, sweet potatoes, carrots, asparagus, cherries, apples, blueberries, strawberries, and millet

- **Animal Protein:** all seafood, meat, chicken, turkey, (all fowl) eggs, pasture-raised meats, and wild-caught fish

- **Fats:** such as those found in avocados, butter, and olive oil

- **Fructose-containing foods:** raw honey, citrus fruits, berries, and pineapple

- **Best starches:** Japanese and purple sweet potatoes (better when they are pressured cooked)

Reducing lectin content of a diet

The lectin content of food can be reduced either by pressure cooking or, for beans, boiling and soaking.

If you have chronic inflammation, are experiencing unexplained weight gain, or have a problem with indigestion, trying an elimination diet may help you manage your health issues.

Benefits of a Lectin Free Diet

- **It can help you to avoid potentially toxic foods**

Beans, such as kidney beans, have been found to be toxic to people due to their very high lectin levels.

- **It might reduce peptic ulcers**

Lectin spikes bacterial growth in the small intestine and strips away the mucous defense layer, increasing the risk of peptic ulcers.

- **It may help you avoid damage to your digestive tract**

Recent research conducted on rats has shown that lectin can disrupt digestion and cause intestinal damage if eaten in large quantities over a long period.

- **It helps reduce cardiovascular diseases**

Lectin-free diets can help reduce the signs and symptoms of **cardiovascular diseases and metabolic syndrome.**

These are a group of conditions indicated by increased blood pressure, high blood-sugar levels, excess body fat around the waist, and abnormal cholesterol levels.

- **It helps you lose weight**

Eating a lectin-free diet **helps you reduce your weight** even when you continue to eat high-calorie foods. This is because you are not storing it as fat anymore.

Lectin-Free Pantry Staples and Seasonings

In certain ways, lectins negatively affect the health of many individuals. This can vary from the risks of chronic diseases to complications in the digestive system and clustering of red blood cells. So when trying to go lectin-free, what should be the staples found in the pantry at home?

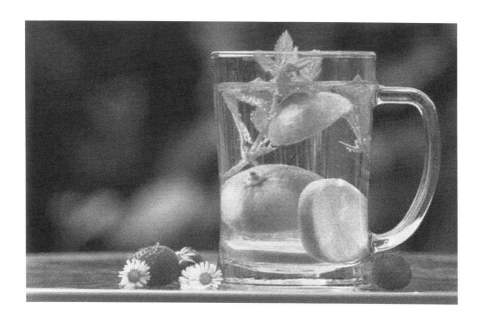

According to studies, individuals who want to effectively lessen and limit their lectin consumption must consume these **recommended food items:**

- A2 milk
- Sweet potatoes
- Pasture-raised meats
- Leafy green vegetables
- Cruciferous vegetables such as broccoli and brussels sprouts
- Onions
- Garlic
- Asparagus
- Celery

- Olives and extra virgin olive oil
- Mushrooms
- Avocados

Here are some lectin-free foods:

- Grass-fed meat
- Pastured poultry
- Wild-caught seafood
- Seeds and nuts (except peanuts, pumpkin seeds, chia, sunflower seeds, and cashews)
- Ghee, olive oil, and European butter
- Stevia
- Dark chocolate that is at least 72% cacao

Suggested substitutions:

- Aminos instead of soy sauce
- Almond flour instead of wheat flour
- Duke's mayonnaise, instead of regular mayonnaise
- Ghee, instead of conventional butter
- No-Ketchup BBQ sauce instead of regular BBQ sauce

- Unsweetened coconut milk and unsweetened almond milk instead of milk
- Stevia instead of sugar
- Arrowroot powder instead of cornstarch

What is an Instant Pot?

An instant pot is a multi-function, countertop pressure cooker. It can function as a slow cooker, rice cooker, steamer, and warmer. Models that are currently out on the market have pasteurization, browning, sautéing, and yogurt-making functions.

This kitchen tool comes in three general capacities and sizes: five, six, and eight quarts. With bigger capacity models, homemade yogurt or steamed bread can be achieved. This can also be used for pasteurizing milk and certain cheeses, and for making broths, stews, and soups for large groups and putting up for later.

Instant Pot is a whisper-quiet tool that cooks food under pressure and is extremely versatile. Whether it is a lectin-free diet or not, an instant pot can correctly prepare foods in a jiff. With a wide range of programmable settings, many foods can be easily prepared.

Advantages of Instant Pot

It is a multi-function tool which can be left alone to do the cooking for you; all that needs to be done are the following:

- Prepare the ingredients before cooking and place into the machine;
- Make sure that the lid is twisted and locked to seal the steamer valve;
- Set it to the desired function that includes, pressure, steam, and time;
- Wait for everything to be cooked;
- Take note of the pressure to be released;
- Add remaining ingredients (if there's any);
- Garnish, serve, and eat!

1. An instant pot has a **"keep warm" function** that automatically turns on when the cooking process has ended. Meals can be cooked 75% to 100% faster than conventional methods.

2. You can **make meals in advance**—make meals in the morning and go home to a warm supper, or, set up the instant pot at night before going to bed so that breakfast is ready in the morning.

3. **Everything is automatic**. Just read the manufacturer's guide for the equipment and learn how versatile it can be for you to cook different lectin-free meals.

4. **It preserves nutrients**—since the machine uses pressure in cooking, the heat is evenly distributed inside the device. The addition of too much water can be avoided to generate steam and cook food. Because food is cooked in a sealed environment, vitamins and minerals are not lost by water or steam.

5. You can enjoy **mess-free cooking.** Since this is a one-pot cooking machine, so preparation and cooking efforts are lessened.

Soups

Chicken Kale Soup

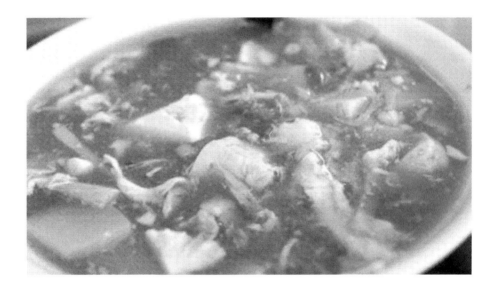

Prep Time: 35 minutes

Servings: 6

Ingredients

- 2 pounds boneless, skinless chicken breasts or chicken thighs
- ½ cup olive oil, avocado oil, coconut oil, or ghee
- ¼ cup lemon juice
- 1 teaspoon lemon zest
- 1 yellow onion, finely chopped

- 2 cloves garlic, minced
- 4 cups homemade, low-sodium chicken broth
- 1 large bunch kale, stemmed and roughly chopped
- 2 tablespoons organic taco seasoning
- 1 teaspoon smoked paprika or regular paprika
- pinch of salt, pepper
- fresh green onions, diced

Method

1. Set your Instant Pot to "Sauté" mode. Add 1 tablespoon olive oil.
2. Once hot, add chicken. Sear 2 minutes per side, until brown.
3. To your blender add chicken broth, onion, garlic, and remaining olive oil. Blend until smooth. Pour into Instant Pot.
4. Stir in lemon juice, lemon zest, kale, taco seasoning, paprika, salt, and pepper.
5. Lock, seal lid, and press the "Manual" button. Cook on HIGH for 10 minutes.
6. When done, naturally release pressure for 10 minutes, then quick release pressure.
7. Serve in bowls, garnish with fresh green onion.

Nutrition information per serving

Calories: 273

Fat: 22.32g, Carbohydrates: 2.4g, Dietary Fiber: 1.1g, Protein: 15.3g

Chicken Turmeric Soup

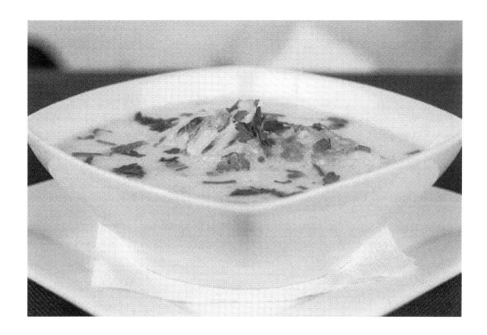

Prep Time: 30 minutes

Servings: 4

Ingredients

- 1½ pounds boneless, skinless chicken breasts or chicken thighs
- 2 tablespoons olive oil, coconut oil, or ghee
- 1 yellow onion, finely chopped
- 2 cloves garlic, minced
- 1 cup cauliflower florets
- 1 cup broccoli florets

- 1 cup carrots, finely chopped
- 1 cup celery stalks, finely chopped
- 4 cups organic, homemade, low-sodium vegetable, bone, or chicken broth
- 1 bay leaf
- 1 teaspoon fresh ginger, grated
- 2 cups Swiss chard, stemmed and roughly chopped
- ½ cup unsweetened coconut cream
- 3 teaspoons turmeric powder
- 1 teaspoon cumin powder
- pinch each of cayenne pepper, salt, black pepper
- fresh cilantro
- lemon wedges

Method

1. Set your Instant Pot to "Sauté" mode. Add olive oil.
2. Once hot, add chicken. Sear 2 minutes per side, until brown. Remove and set aside.
3. Add onion, ginger, and garlic to Instant Pot. Sauté until softened.
4. Add cauliflower, broccoli, carrots, and celery. Sauté for 1 minute. Return chicken to pot. Add broth, bay leaf, turmeric powder, cumin powder, cayenne pepper, salt, and pepper. Stir to combine. Lock, seal lid, and press the "Manual" button. Cook on HIGH for 8 minutes.

5. When done, naturally release pressure for 5 minutes. Remove the lid. Remove bay leaf.
6. Stir in coconut cream and Swiss chard until chard wilts.
7. Ladle soup into bowls. Garnish with fresh cilantro and lemon wedges. Serve.

Nutrition information per serving

- **Calories: 428**
- Fat: 42.65g
- Carbohydrates: 11.71g
- Dietary Fiber: 3.4g
- Protein: 42.53g

Thai Broccoli and Beef Soup

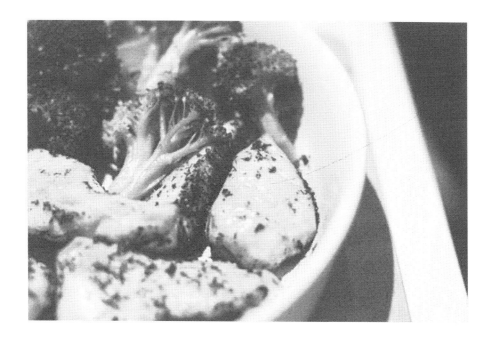

Prep Time: 20 minutes

Servings: 4

Ingredients

- 1 pound lean, grass-fed ground beef
- 2 large heads broccoli, chopped into florets
- 1 cup unsweetened coconut cream
- ⅓ cup fresh cilantro, finely chopped
- 2 tablespoons organic Thai green curry paste
- 2 tablespoons olive oil
- 1 medium-sized onion, finely chopped
- 2-inch piece of ginger, peeled and minced

- 2 cloves garlic, minced
- 3 tablespoons low-sodium coconut aminos
- 1 teaspoon organic fish sauce
- 4 cups homemade, low-sodium chicken or beef broth
- pinch of salt, pepper

Method

1. Set your Instant Pot to "Sauté" mode and add olive oil.
2. Once hot, add onions. Sauté for 2 to 4 minutes.
3. Add ginger, garlic, and green curry paste to Instant Pot. Cook for 1 minute.
4. Add ground beef. Cook until no longer pink. Stir in coconut aminos, salt, pepper, and fish sauce. Add broth to Instant Pot.
5. Lock, seal lid, and press the "Manual" button. Cook on HIGH for 8 minutes.
6. When done, naturally release pressure for 5 minutes. Carefully remove the lid.
7. Stir in broccoli florets. Allow to heat through for a couple of minutes.
8. Stir in coconut cream. Season to taste and serve in bowls.

Nutrition information per serving

Calories: 422

Fat: 34.33g, Carbohydrates: 5.6g, Dietary Fiber: 2.9g, Protein: 27.35g

Roasted Garlic Soup

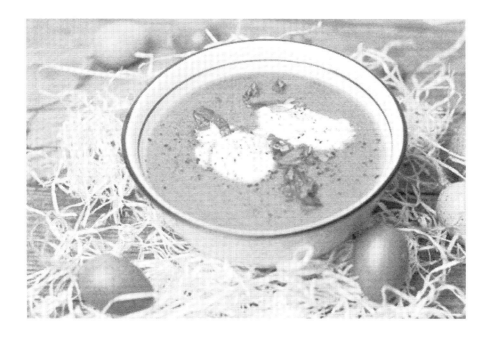

Prep Time: 35 minutes

Servings: 6

Ingredients

- 2 bulbs of garlic (around 20 garlic cloves)
- 1 large cauliflower head, finely chopped
- ¼ cup ghee or non-dairy butter
- 3 medium shallots or onions, finely chopped
- 6 cups homemade, low-sodium vegetable broth
- pinch of salt, pepper
- 1 cup unsweetened coconut cream

Method

1. Set your Instant Pot to "Sauté" mode. Add the ghee.
2. Once hot, add onions and garlic. Sauté for 3 to 5 minutes.
3. Add cauliflower, vegetable broth, salt, and pepper.
4. Lock, seal lid, and press the "Manual" button. Cook on HIGH for 30 minutes.
5. When done, quick release pressure and carefully remove the lid.
6. Use an immersion blender to puree the soup until smooth.
7. Stir in coconut cream. Season to taste and serve in bowls.

Nutrition information per serving

- **Calories: 156**
- Fat: 14.05g
- Carbohydrates: 8.17g
- Dietary Fiber: 2g
- Protein: 2.94g

Hamburger Vegetable Soup

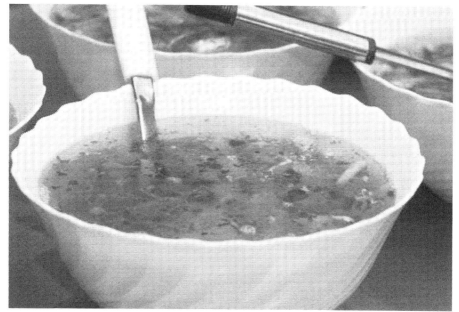

Prep Time: 19 minutes

Servings: 10

Ingredients

- 1 pound extra-lean grass-fed ground beef
- 2 cups fresh green cabbage, shredded
- 2 cups fresh red cabbage, shredded
- 2 tablespoons olive oil
- 1 medium-sized red onion, finely chopped
- 4 cloves garlic, minced
- 3 fresh celery ribs, finely chopped
- 3 fresh carrots, peeled and finely chopped

- 1 large sweet potato, peeled and cubed
- 1 teaspoon cider vinegar
- 1 teaspoon stevia
- 1 cup pureed pumpkin
- 4 cups homemade, low-sodium chicken broth
- pinch of salt, pepper

Method

1. Set your Instant Pot to "Sauté" mode. Add the olive oil.
2. Once hot, add onions and garlic. Sauté for 2 minutes, until soft.
3. Add ground beef. Cook until no longer pink.
4. Add celery, carrots, and cubed sweet potatoes. Cook for 1 minute.
5. Stir in pureed pumpkin, chicken broth, green cabbage, red cabbage, cider vinegar, stevia, salt, and black pepper.
6. Lock, seal lid, and press the "Manual" button. Cook on HIGH for 9 minutes.
7. When done, naturally release pressure for 5 minutes, then quick release. Remove lid.
8. Stir the soup. Season to taste and serve in bowls.

Nutrition information per serving

Calories: 132

Fat: 5.3g, Carbohydrates: 7.3g, Dietary Fiber: 3.9g, Protein: 14.3g

Vegetable Recipes

Sesame Bok Choy Platter

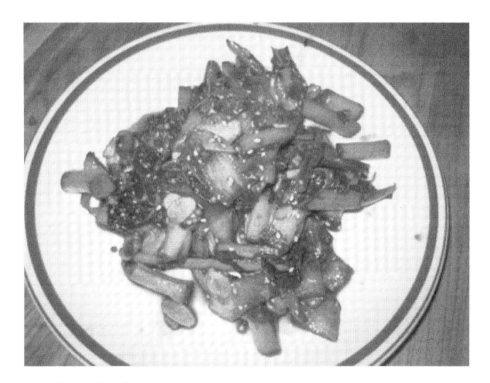

Prep Time: 5 minutes

Cooking Time: 4 minutes

Servings: 4

Ingredients

- 1 cup water
- 1 medium head bok choy, leaves separated

- 1 teaspoon coconut aminos
- ½ teaspoon sesame oil
- 2 teaspoons sesame seeds
- Salt and pepper as needed

Method

1. Add water to Instant Pot
2. Insert steamer rack
3. Stack bok choy on steamer rack with the largest/thickest leaves on the bottom
4. Lock, seal lid and cook on HIGH pressure for 4 minutes
5. Once done, quick release pressure
6. Transfer bok choy to a large bowl and toss with coconut aminos, sesame oil, and sesame seeds
7. Season with salt and pepper
8. Enjoy!

Nutrition information per serving

Calories: 54

Total Fat: 0g, Saturated Fat: 0g, Cholesterol: 0mg, Sodium: 246mg, Total Carbs: 5g, Fiber: 2g, Sugar: 2g, Protein: 3, Potassium: 359mg

Cool Instant Pot Broccoli

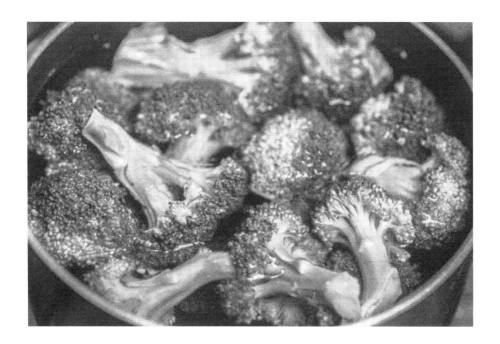

Servings: 2

Prep Time: 3 minutes

Cooking Time: 4 minutes

Ingredients

- 1 medium head broccoli, chopped into florets
- Salt and pepper as needed
- ¾ cup water

Method

1. Add ¾ cup of water to your Instant Pot
2. Chop broccoli head into florets
3. Place steamer rack in your Instant Pot and add the florets
4. Lock lid and cook on HIGH pressure for 2 minutes
5. Release pressure naturally over 10 minutes
6. Season to taste with salt and pepper
7. Enjoy!

Nutrition information per serving

- **Calories: 33**
- Total Fat: 3g
- Saturated Fat: 1g
- Cholesterol: 0mg
- Sodium: 188mg
- Total Carbs: 2g
- Fiber: 3g
- Sugar: 2g
- Protein: 1g
- Potassium: 307mg

Awesome Parsnips and Chive Soup

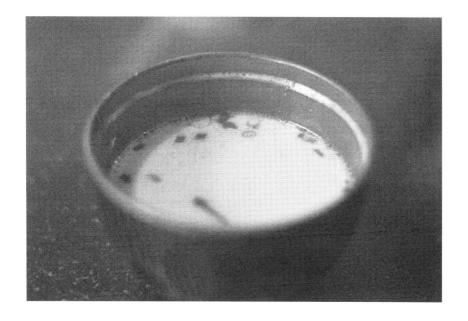

Servings: 4-6

Prep Time: 10 minutes

Cooking Time: 10 minutes

Ingredients

- 3 pounds parsnips, trimmed and peeled
- 3 cloves garlic
- ½ cup raw cashews
- 6 cups vegetable broth
- ¼ cup olive oil

- juice of half lemon
- 1 teaspoon salt
- pinch of pepper
- ¼ cup fresh chives, more for garnish

Method

1. Add parsnips, raw cashews, garlic, and broth to your Instant Pot
2. Set your Instant Pot to "Sauté" mode and let it come to a boil
3. Cancel Saute and lock lid
4. Cook on HIGH pressure for 10 minutes
5. Quick release the pressure
6. Remove lid and blend soup using an immersion blender
7. If you want a thinner soup, add ½ cup more broth
8. Season with lemon juice, pepper, chives, and salt
9. Serve with a topping of more chives and a drizzle of olive oil
10. Enjoy!

Nutrition information per serving

Calories: 289

Total Fat: 13g, Saturated Fat: 2g, Cholesterol: 0mg, Sodium: 1098mg, Total Carbs: 35g, Fiber: 12g, Sugar: 11g, Protein: 4g, Potassium: 4mg

Subtle Braised Cabbage

Servings: 6

Prep Time: 5 minutes

Cooking Time: 3 minutes

Ingredients

- 3 slices bacon
- 1 tablespoon clarified butter
- 1 small head green cabbage, cored, quartered, and cut into ½ inch strips
- 1 cup vegetable broth
- salt
- fresh ground black pepper

Method

1. Set your Instant Pot to "Sauté" mode and add bacon in one layer.
2. Saute for 5 minutes or until crisp, making sure to flip halfway through.
3. Remove bacon and cut into pieces.
4. Add more clarified butter and let it heat.
5. Add cabbage, broth, and cooked bacon.

6. Season with salt and pepper.
7. Lock lid and cook on HIGH pressure for 3 minutes.
8. Quick release pressure.
9. Serve and enjoy!

Nutrition information per serving

- **Calories: 70**
- Total Fat: 10g
- Saturated Fat: 2g
- Cholesterol: 20mg
- Sodium: 263mg
- Total Carbs: 7g
- Fiber: 3g
- Sugar: 3g
- Protein: 3g
- Potassium: 293mg

Delicious Bowl of Mushrooms

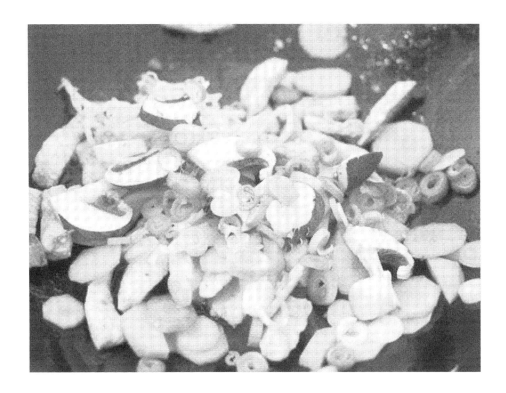

Servings: 4

Prep Time: 10 minutes

Cooking Time: 20 minutes

Ingredients

- 8 cups vegetable stock
- 1 pound baby Bella mushrooms, sliced
- 1 medium onion, diced
- 2 celery stalks, diced

- 2 carrots, diced
- 4 cloves garlic, chopped
- 4 sprigs thyme
- 1 sprig sage
- 1 teaspoon salt
- ¼ teaspoon freshly ground pepper
- ¼ teaspoon garlic powder

Method

1. Add listed ingredients to your Instant Pot
2. Stir to combine and lock lid
3. Cook on HIGH pressure for 10 minutes
4. Once the cooking is complete, release the pressure naturally over 10 minutes
5. Serve and enjoy!

Nutrition information per serving

Calories: 114

Total Fat: 5g, Saturated Fat: 1g, Cholesterol: 0mg, Sodium: 648mg, Total Carbs: 15g, Fiber: 3g, Sugar: 8g, Protein: 7g, Potassium: 701mg

Yummy Roasted Artichoke Platter

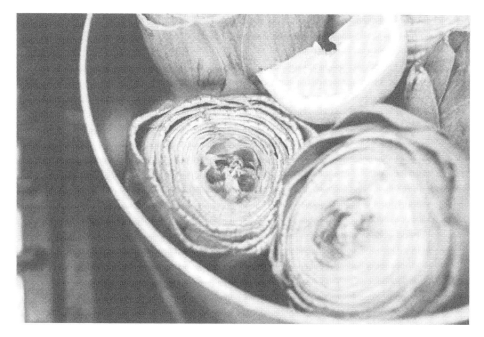

Servings: 4

Prep Time: 10 minutes

Cooking Time: 27 minutes

Ingredients

- 2 whole artichokes
- 3 lemons
- 2 cloves garlic, peeled and sliced
- 3 tablespoons olive oil
- Flavored vinegar
- black pepper as needed

Method

1. Wash your artichokes thoroughly under cold water
2. Trim ½ inch from the top and cut stem to about ½ inch length
3. Trim the artichokes by cutting off thorny parts and tough leaves
4. Rub the cut areas with lemon
5. Poke garlic slivers between the artichoke leaves
6. Place steamer rack in Instant Pot
7. Place prepared artichokes in the steamer rack
8. Lock lid and cook on HIGH pressure for 7 minutes
9. Release pressure naturally over 10 minutes
10. Transfer artichokes to cutting board and let them rest
11. Cut the artichokes in half lengthwise and remove the purple-white center
12. Preheat your oven to 400°F
13. Make a dressing by blending olive oil with the juice of one lemon
14. Pour the mix over your artichoke halves and sprinkle with pepper and vinegar
15. Preheat a cast iron skillet in the oven for 5 minutes
16. Drizzle a few teaspoons of oil in the heated skillet and add marinated artichoke halves
17. Brush with lemon juice and olive oil dressing
18. Cut another lemon into quarters and nestle between the halves
19. Roast for 20-25 minutes until the artichokes are browned
20. Enjoy!

Nutrition information per serving

Calories: 268

Total Fat: 4g, Saturated Fat: 1g, Cholesterol: 0mg, Sodium: 570mg, Total Carbs: 45g, Fiber: 2g, Sugar: 4g, Protein: 14g, Potassium: 757mg

Feisty Pot of Brussels Sprouts

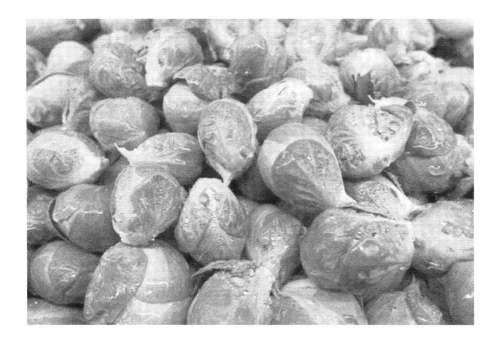

Servings: 4

Prep Time: 10 minutes

Cooking Time: 5 minutes

Ingredients

- 2 pounds Brussels sprouts, halved
- ¼ cup coconut aminos
- 2 tablespoons sriracha sauce (lectin-free variety)
- 1 tablespoon vinegar
- 2 tablespoons olive oil

- 1 tablespoon almonds, chopped
- 1 teaspoon red pepper flakes
- 2 teaspoons garlic powder
- 1 teaspoon onion powder
- 1 tablespoon smoked paprika
- ½ teaspoon cayenne pepper
- salt and pepper as needed

Method

1. Set your Instant Pot to "Sauté" mode and add almonds
2. Toast them for briefly
3. Add the remaining ingredients (except the Brussels sprouts) to a bowl and give it a gentle toss to mix
4. Add the Brussels sprouts to the pot along with the prepped mixture
5. Stir to combine thoroughly and lock lid
6. Cook on HIGH pressure for 3 minutes
7. Release the pressure naturally and serve!

Nutrition information per serving

Calories: 84

Total Fat: 7g, Saturated Fat: 5g, Cholesterol: 19mg, Sodium: 183mg, Total Carbs: 5g, Fiber: 2g, Sugar: 2g, Protein: 2g, Potassium: 271mg

Creamy Leek and Broccoli Soup

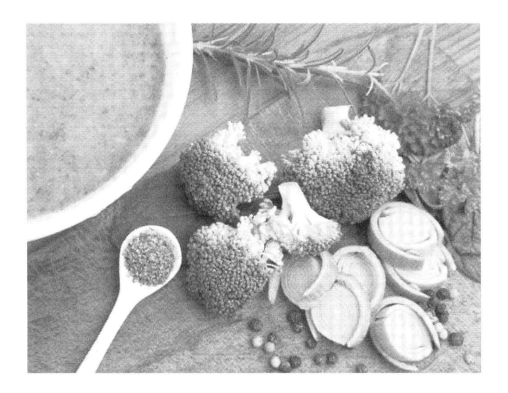

Servings: 2

Prep Time: 10 minutes

Cooking Time: 8 minutes

Ingredients

- 2 tablespoons ghee
- 3 medium leeks, white parts only
- 2 shallots, chopped
- 1 large head broccoli, cut into florets

- 4 cups vegetable broth
- 1 cup unsweetened coconut milk
- pepper and salt as needed
- ¼ cup walnuts, toasted
- ¼ cup coconut cream

Method

1. Set your Instant Pot to "Sauté" mode and add ghee, allow the ghee to melt
2. Add leeks and shallots and cook for 4 to 6 minutes
3. Add broccoli and saute for 5 to 6 minutes
4. Add vegetable broth and coconut milk and stir to combine
5. Lock lid and cook on HIGH pressure for 5 minutes
6. Release the pressure over 10 minutes
7. Open lid and puree using an immersion blender
8. Serve with a garnish of walnuts and a drizzle of coconut cream
9. Enjoy!

Nutrition information per serving

Calories: 194

Total Fat: 8g, Saturated Fat: 9g, Cholesterol: 0m, Sodium: 674mg, Total Carbs: 29g, Fiber: 7g, Sugar: 5g, Protein: 7g, Potassium: 902mg

Garlic and Broccoli Mash

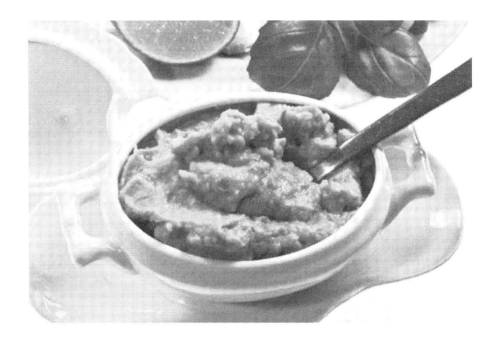

Servings: 4

Prep Time: 3 minutes

Cooking Time: 12 minutes

Ingredients

- 2 whole broccoli heads, cut into florets
- ½ cup water
- 6 cloves garlic, minced
- 1 tablespoon olive oil
- 1 tablespoon white wine vinegar

- salt as needed

Method

1. Place steamer rack in your Instant Pot and add florets to the rack.
2. Add ½ cup water.
3. Lock the lid and cook on LOW for 10 minutes.
4. Quick release.
5. Cool broccoli by transferring to an ice bath.
6. Remove water and Set your Instant Pot to "Sauté" mode.
7. Add olive oil and minced garlic.
8. Saute for 25-30 seconds then add the broccoli and white wine vinegar.
9. Season with a bit of salt and stir for 30 seconds.
10. Enjoy!

Nutrition information per serving

Calories: 101

Total Fat: 8g, Saturated Fat: 1g, Cholesterol: 0mg, Sodium: 57mg, Total Carbs: 6g, Fiber: 5g, Sugar: 1g, Protein: 6g, Potassium: 347mg

Healthy Carrot Soup

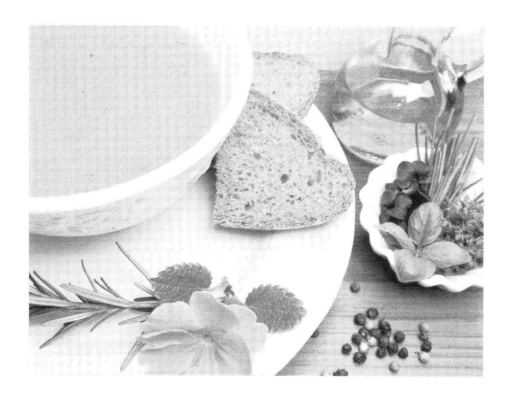

Servings: 4

Prep Time: 10 minutes

Cooking Time: 15 minutes

Ingredients

- 1 tablespoon ghee
- ½ yellow onion, chopped
- 3 cloves garlic, minced
- 1 tablespoon curry powder

- 1 teaspoon cayenne pepper
- 1½ cups vegetable broth
- 8-10 large carrots, peeled and chopped
- 1 14-ounce can unsweetened coconut milk

Method

1. Set your Instant Pot to "Sauté" mode and add ghee, let the ghee melt
2. Add onion and garlic and cook for 3 to 5 minutes
3. Add all remaining ingredients except coconut milk
4. Give it a nice stir
5. Lock lid and cook on HIGH pressure for 15 minutes
6. Release pressure naturally over 10 minutes
7. Puree the mix using an immersion blender
8. Stir in unsweetened coconut milk and adjust seasoning
9. Serve and enjoy!

Nutrition information per serving

Calories: 102

Total Fat: 1g, Saturated Fat: 0g, Cholesterol: 0mg, Sodium: 196mg, Total Carbs: 35g, Fiber: 10g, Sugar: 20g, Protein: 2g, Potassium: 1026mg

Seafood Recipes

Fantastic Ginger Tilapia

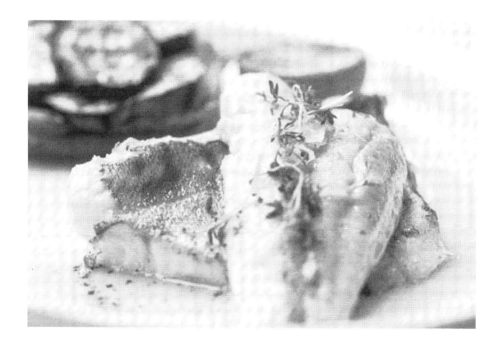

Servings: 4

Prep Time: 10 minutes + 2 hours marinating time

Cooking Time: 5 minutes

Ingredients

- 1 pound tilapia fillets
- 3 tablespoons low-sodium coconut aminos
- 2 tablespoons white vinegar
- 2 cloves garlic, minced
- pinch of salt and pepper
- 1 tablespoon olive oil
- 2 tablespoons fresh ginger, julienned
- ¼ cup fresh scallions, julienned
- ¼ cup fresh cilantro, chopped

Method

1. Add coconut aminos, minced garlic, white vinegar, salt, and pepper to a large bowl and stir to combine.
2. Add tilapia to the bowl and toss gently, carefully spooning the sauce over the fish to ensure that it is coated well.
3. Allow fish to marinate for 2 hours in the refrigerator.
4. Add 2 cups water to your Instant Pot.
5. Place steamer rack in Instant Pot and transfer the marinated fillets to the steamer rack.
6. Lock, seal lid, and cook on LOW Pressure for 2 minutes.
7. Quick release the pressure.
8. Transfer fillets to serving the dish and discard water from the pot.

9. Set your Instant Pot to "Sauté" mode and add olive oil, allow the oil to heat up
10. Add julienned ginger and sauté for a few seconds
11. Add scallions and cilantro and sauté for 2 minutes
12. Stir in marinade and let it heat up
13. Spoon all of the sauce over the fish and serve
14. Enjoy!

Nutrition information per serving

- **Calories: 176**
- Total Fat: 6g
- Saturated Fat: 1g
- Cholesterol: 73mg
- Sodium: 958mg
- Total Carbs: 5g
- Fiber: 1g
- Sugar: 1g
- Protein: 25g
- Potassium: 589mg

Pepper Lemon Salmon

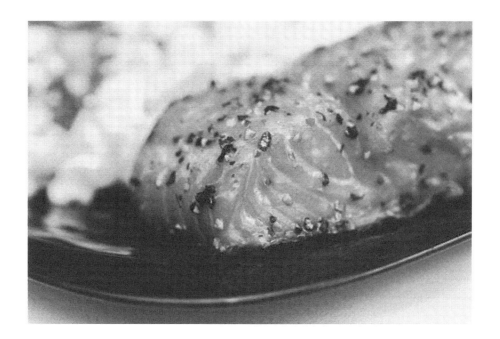

Servings: 3

Prep Time: 5 minutes

Cooking Time: 6 minutes

Ingredients

- ¾ cup water
- few sprigs of parsley, basil, tarragon
- 1 pound salmon, skin on
- 3 teaspoons ghee
- ¼ teaspoon salt

- ½ teaspoon pepper
- ½ lemon, thinly sliced
- 1 whole carrot, julienned

Method

1. Set your Instant Pot to "Sauté" mode and add water and herbs
2. Insert steamer rack in Instant Pot and place salmon in the rack
3. Drizzle ghee on top of salmon
4. Season with salt and pepper
5. Cover with lemon slices
6. Lock lid and cook on HIGH pressure for 3 minutes
7. Once done, release pressure naturally over 10 minutes
8. Transfer salmon to a serving platter
9. Discard water and Set your Instant Pot to "Sauté" mode
10. Add vegetables and cook for 1 to 2 minutes
11. Serve vegetables with the salmon
12. Enjoy!

Nutrition information per serving

Calories: 464

Total Fat: 34g, Saturated Fat: 10g, Cholesterol: 110mg, Sodium: 529mg, Total Carbs: 3g, Fiber: 1g, Sugar: 2g, Protein: 34g, Potassium: 694mg

Gentle Crab Legs

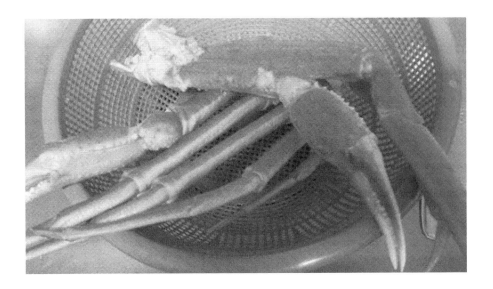

Servings: 4

Prep Time: 5 minutes

Cooking Time: 5 minutes

Ingredients

- 2 pounds crab legs
- 1 cup water
- 1 cup white wine vinegar
- 1 lemon sliced up into wedges

Method

1. Add water and vinegar to your Instant Pot.
2. Add crab legs.
3. Lock up the lid and cook on HIGH pressure for 7 minutes.
4. Release the pressure naturally over 10 minutes.
5. Open the lid and serve with lemon wedges.
6. Enjoy!

Nutrition information per serving

- **Calories: 191**
- Total Fat: 1g
- Saturated Fat: 0g
- Cholesterol: 95mg
- Sodium: 1896mg
- Total Carbs: 0g
- Fiber: 0g
- Sugar: 0g
- Protein: 4g
- Potassium: 463mg

Slightly Spicy Chili Salmon

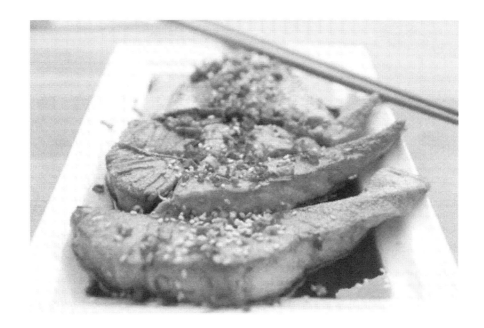

Servings: 6

Prep Time: 5 minutes

Cooking Time: 5 minutes

Ingredients

- 1 pound salmon fillet cut into 4 pieces
- Salt as needed
- Pepper as needed
- 1 tablespoon chili powder
- 1 teaspoon ground cumin

- 1 teaspoon garlic powder
- 1 avocado, diced
- 1 teaspoon lime juice
- cilantro for garnish, chopped

Method

1. Add 1 cup of water to your Instant Pot and insert steamer rack.
2. To a small bowl add ground cumin, garlic powder, and chili powder, mix well.
3. Rub fillets with mixture and transfer to the steamer rack.
4. Lock lid and cook on HIGH pressure for 2 minutes.
5. Naturally, release the pressure over 10 minutes.
6. Top with avocado and serve.
7. Enjoy!

Nutrition information per serving

Calories: 125

Total Fat: 1g, Saturated Fat: 0g, Cholesterol: 0mg, Sodium: 213mg, Total Carbs: 22g, Fiber: 2g, Sugar: 4g, Protein: 30g, Potassium: 302mg

Juicy Coconut Fish Curry

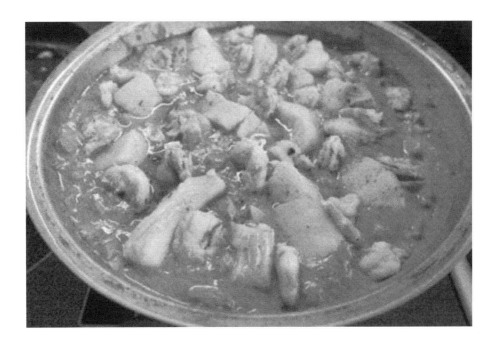

Servings: 4

Prep Time: 5 minutes

Cooking Time: 5 minutes

Ingredients

- 1 can coconut milk
- juice of 1 lime
- 1 tablespoon red curry paste
- 1 teaspoon fish sauce
- 1 teaspoon coconut aminos
- 1 teaspoon date paste

- 2 teaspoons Sriracha
- 2 cloves garlic, minced
- 1 teaspoon ground turmeric
- 1 teaspoon ground ginger
- ½ teaspoon sea salt
- ½ teaspoon white pepper
- 1 pound sea bass or cod, cut into 1-inch cubes
- ¼ cup fresh cilantro, chopped
- 3 lime wedges

Method

1. To a large bowl, add coconut milk, red curry paste, lime juice, fish sauce, date paste, garlic sriracha, aminos, ginger, white pepper, turmeric, and sea salt, give it a nice mix
2. Place sea bass/cod in the bottom of your Instant Pot
3. Pour coconut milk over fish and lock lid
4. Cook on HIGH pressure for 3 minutes
5. Quick release pressure
6. Transfer fish and broth to your serving platter
7. Garnish with chopped cilantro
8. Serve and enjoy!

Nutrition information per serving

Calories: 278, Total Fat: 18 g, Saturated Fat: 12g, Cholesterol: 57mg, Sodium: 399mg, Total Carbs: 7g, Fiber: 1g, Sugar: 2g, Protein: 25g

Pork Recipes

Hearty Lemon and Artichoke Pork Chops

Servings: 4

Prep Time: 5 minutes

Cooking Time: 15 minutes

Ingredients

- 3 ounces bacon, diced
- 4 ½-inch thick bone-in pork chops
- 2 teaspoons ground black pepper
- 1 shallot, minced
- 1 teaspoon lemon zest
- 3 cloves garlic, minced
- 1 teaspoon dried rosemary
- 1 cup chicken broth
- 1 9-ounce package frozen artichoke heart quarters

Method

1. Set your Instant Pot to "Sauté" mode and add bacon
2. Cook for 5 minutes until the fat is rendered and the bacon is crispy
3. Transfer the bacon to a plate
4. Season the chops with pepper and salt and transfer to your Instant Pot
5. Brown the chops, do in batches if needed
6. Add shallots and cook for 1 minute
7. Add lemon zest, rosemary, and garlic and cook until fragrant
8. Add chicken broth, artichokes, cooked bacon and stir
9. Nestle the chops back to the bottom of the Instant Pot
10. Lock the lid and cook on HIGH pressure on MEAT/STEW setting for 15 minutes
11. Perform a quick release
12. Open the lid and season with salt and pepper
13. Serve with the lemon artichoke sauce
14. Enjoy!

Nutrition information per serving
Calories: 286

Total Fat: 26g, Saturated Fat: 6g, Cholesterol: 137mg, Sodium: 110mg, Total Carbs: 5g, Fiber: 0g, Sugar: 0g, Protein: 41g

Tender Soft Pineapple Pork Chops

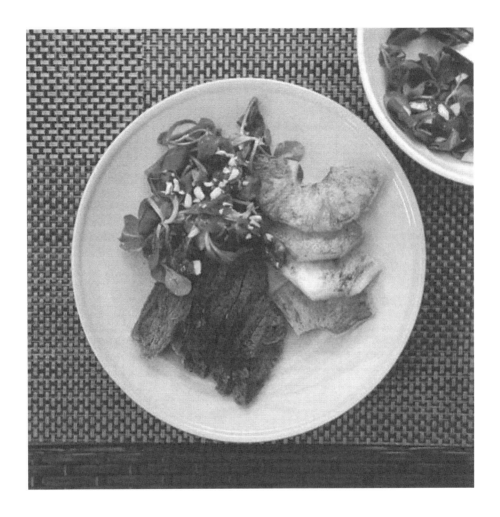

Servings: 4

Prep Time: 10 minutes

Cooking Time: 25 minutes

Ingredients

- 6 thin-cut pork chops
- balsamic glaze
- seasoning of your choice (for pork chops)
- olive oil as needed
- cubed pineapple

Method

1. Season the chops well on all sides.
2. Set your Instant Pot to "Sauté" mode and drizzle olive oil into the bottom of the pot.
3. Allow it to heat for a minute.
4. Add pork chops to the pot and sear well on both sides.
5. Remove the chop and layer them on a steam rack or trivet.
6. Drizzle a bit of glaze over the chops.
7. Spread pineapple chunks over the chops.
8. Add 1 cup of water to the pot and insert the trivet.
9. Lock the lid and cook for 25 minutes on HIGH pressure.
10. Naturally release the pressure and remove the chops.
11. Garnish with more glaze and pineapples and enjoy!

Nutrition information per serving

Calories: 621

Total Fat: 15g, Saturated Fat: 7g, Cholesterol: 137mg, Sodium: 913mg, Total Carbs: 25g, Fiber: 4g, Sugar: 16g, Protein: 24g

Onion Pork Bliss

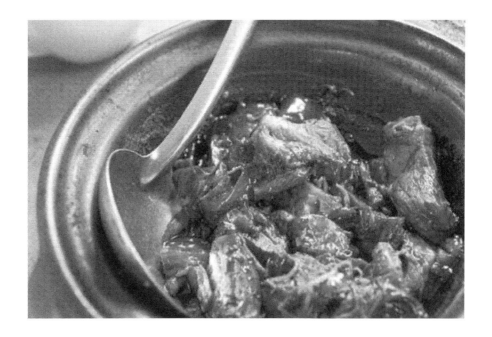

Servings: 4

Prep Time: 10 minutes

Cooking Time: 40 minutes

Ingredients

- 1 onion, chopped
- 2 pounds pork shoulder
- 2 cups beef broth
- ½ cup water
- juice of 2 limes

- 1 teaspoon oregano
- 1 teaspoon cumin
- 2 teaspoons garlic, minced
- 1 tablespoon olive oil
- 1 jalapeno, deseeded, peeled and diced

Method

1. Set your Instant Pot to "Sauté" mode and add oil; let it heat up.
2. Add pork and sear on all sides until browned.
3. Add rest of the ingredients and stir.
4. Lock lid and cook on HIGH pressure for 30 minutes.
5. Release pressure naturally over 10 minutes.
6. Open lid and shred meat with two forks.
7. Leave on SAUTE mode and cook for a few minutes more if you prefer a thicker sauce.
8. Serve and enjoy!

Nutrition information per serving

Calories: 412

Total Fat: 24g, Saturated Fat: 9, Cholesterol: 150mg, Sodium: 211mg, Total Carbs: 2g, Fiber: 2g, Sugar: 0g, Protein: 344, Potassium: 712mg

Easy Jamaican Pork

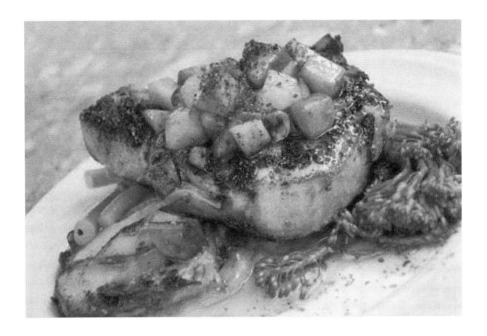

Servings: 4

Prep Time: 10 minutes

Cooking Time: 45 minutes

Ingredients

- 1 tablespoon olive oil
- 2 pounds pork shoulder
- 1 cup beef broth
- 2 tablespoons Jamaican Spice Rub

Method

1. Set your pot to SAUTE mode and add oil; let the oil heat up.
2. Add pork and cook until browned well.
3. Add spice rub and broth, and stir.
4. Lock lid and cook on HIGH pressure for 45 minutes.
5. Quickly release pressure.
6. Open lid and shred meat using two forks.
7. Serve and enjoy!

Nutrition information per serving

- **Calories: 888**
- Total Fat: 62g
- Saturated Fat: 21g
- Cholesterol: 242mg
- Sodium: 1514mg
- Total Carbs: 18g
- Fiber: 6g
- Sugar: 6g
- Protein: 64g
- Potassium: 2204mg

Sprouts and Chops Medley

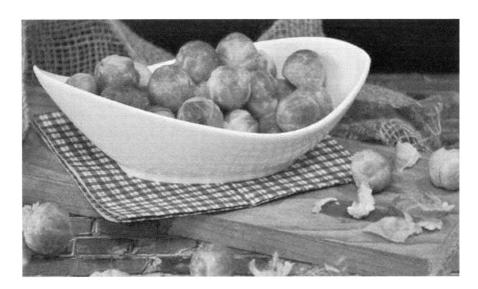

Servings: 4

Prep Time: 10 minutes

Cooking Time: 20 minutes

Ingredients

- 1 tablespoon coconut oil
- 2 cups brussels sprouts
- 4 pork chops, boneless
- ½ teaspoon thyme
- 2 teaspoons garlic cloves
- 1 cup onion, sliced
- 1 tablespoon arrowroot
- 1 cup beef broth

Method

1. Set your pot to SAUTE mode and add coconut oil.
2. Add pork and brown on both sides. Transfer to a plate.
3. Add onions, garlic, and thyme; cook for 1 minute.
4. Add beef broth and return the chops to the pot.
5. Lock lid and cook on HIGH pressure for 15 minutes.
6. Quickly release pressure.
7. Open the lid and add brussels sprouts and pork chops. Close lid and cook on HIGH pressure for 3 minutes.
8. Quickly release pressure.
9. Transfer pork and brussels sprouts to a serving platter.
10. Stir arrowroot in the sauce in the Instant Pot and set the pot to SAUTE mode. Cook until the sauce is thick.
11. Drizzle the sauce over meat.
12. Serve and enjoy!

Nutrition information per serving

Calories: 827

Total Fat: 56g, Saturated Fat: 11g, Cholesterol: 137mg, Sodium: 27mg, Total Carbs: 37g, Fiber: 7g, Sugar: 25g, Protein: 47g,

Potassium: 1277mg

Shredded Cabbage and Bacon

Servings: 4

Prep Time: 10 minutes

Cooking Time: 10 minutes

Ingredients

- 1½ cups beef broth
- 1 pound cabbage, shredded
- 4 large bacon slices, diced
- ½ teaspoon black pepper
- ½ teaspoon salt
- 2 tablespoons clarified butter

Method

1. Set your pot to SAUTE mode and add bacon; cook until crispy.
2. Add butter and heat it up.
3. Add cabbage and season with salt and pepper.
4. Pour in broth.
5. Lock lid and cook on HIGH pressure for 10 minutes.
6. Quickly release pressure.
7. Serve and enjoy!

Nutrition information per serving

Calories: 479

Total Fat: 39g, Saturated Fat:12g, Cholesterol: 57mg, Sodium: 627mg, Total Carbs: 22g, Fiber: 4g, Sugar: 5g, Protein: 13g, Potassium: 802mg

The "Ghee"- Licious Pork Chops

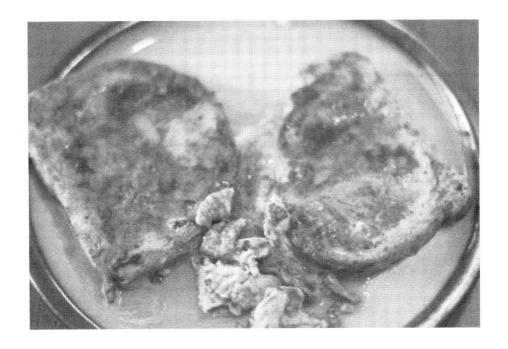

Servings: 4

Prep Time: 10 minutes

Cooking Time: 90 minutes

Ingredients

- 2 tablespoons clarified butter
- 4 thick bone-in pork chops
- ½ teaspoon ground black pepper
- 16 baby carrots, chopped
- 1 tablespoon fresh dill fronds, sliced
- ½ cup white wine vinegar
- ½ cup chicken broth

Method

1. Set your pot to SAUTE mode.
2. Season pork chops with pepper and vinegar.
3. Add pork chops to your pot and cook for 4 minutes.
4. Transfer pork chops to plate and repeat until all chops are browned.
5. Pour 1 tablespoon of clarified butter and add carrots and dill.
6. Cook for 4 minutes.
7. Pour wine vinegar and scrape off any browned bits; bring to a boil.
8. Stir in broth.
9. Return chops and lock lid; cook on HIGH pressure for 8 minutes.
10. Naturally, release pressure over 10 minutes.
11. Serve and enjoy!

Nutrition information per serving

Calories: 459

Total Fat: 24g, Saturated Fat: 10g, Cholesterol: 153mg, Sodium:1546mg, Total Carbs: 13g, Fiber: 2g, Sugar: 10g, Protein: 42g, Potassium: 891mg

Olive Dredged Pork Belly

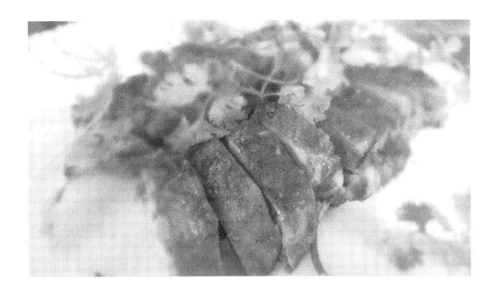

Servings: 4

Prep Time: 10 minutes

Cooking Time: 40 minutes

Ingredients

- 1 pound pork belly
- 3 tablespoons olive oil
- ½ cup white wine vinegar
- 1 rosemary sprig
- 1 garlic clove
- salt and pepper to taste

Method

1. Set your pot to SAUTE mode and add olive oil; let it heat up.
2. Add pork belly and cook 3 minutes each side.
3. Pour in vinegar and place rosemary sprig and garlic inside.
4. Season with salt and pepper.
5. Lock lid and cook on HIGH pressure for 40 minutes.
6. Quickly release pressure.
7. Serve and enjoy!

Nutrition information per serving

- **Calories: 815**
- Total Fat: 46g
- Saturated Fat: 17g
- Cholesterol: 204mg
- Sodium: 222mg
- Total Carbs: 35g
- Fiber: 9g
- Sugar: 12g
- Protein: 63g
- Potassium: 1901mg

Beef Recipes

Exotic Chili and Garlic Beef

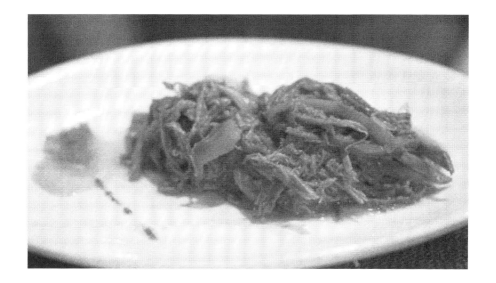

Servings: 4

Prep Time: 10 minutes

Cooking Time: 65 minutes

Ingredients

- 2 pounds chuck roast
- ½ cup water

- 1 onion, sliced
- juice of 2 lemons
- 8 ounces canned green chilies, chopped
- 4 garlic cloves, minced
- 1 tablespoon cumin
- 1 tablespoon oregano
- ½ teaspoon pepper

Method

1. Add the listed ingredients to your Instant Pot.
2. Stir and then lock lid.
3. Cook on HIGH pressure for 60 minutes.
4. Quickly release pressure.
5. Shred the meat using a fork and set your pot to SAUTE mode.
6. Cook for 5 minutes more.
7. Serve and enjoy!

Nutrition information per serving

Calories: 209

Total Fat: 7g, Saturated Fat: 3g, Cholesterol: 95mg, Sodium: 121mg

Total Carbs: 3g, Fiber: 1g, Sugar: 0g, Protein: 33g, Potassium: 606mg

Broccoli and Ginger Beef

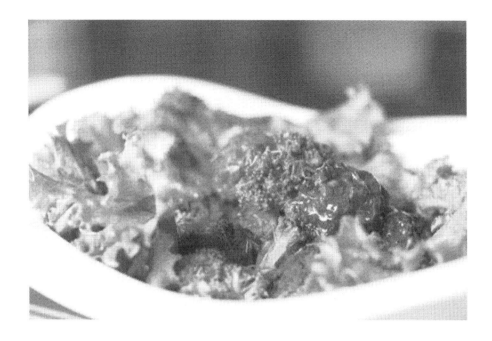

Servings: 4

Prep Time: 10 minutes

Cooking Time: 30 minutes

Ingredients

- 1 onion, quartered
- 12 ounces broccoli florets
- 1 pound beef, chopped
- 2 tablespoons fish sauce
- ¼ cup coconut aminos

- 1 teaspoon garlic, minced
- 1 teaspoon ginger, ground
- ½ teaspoon salt
- ½ teaspoon pepper

Method

1. Add all listed ingredients, except broccoli.
2. Lock lid and cook on MEAT/STEW mode on default settings.
3. Quick release pressure.
4. Open the lid.
5. Stir in broccoli and cook on SAUTE mode for 5 minutes.
6. Serve and enjoy!

Nutrition information per serving

- **Calories: 533**
- Total Fat: 37g
- Saturated Fat: 10g
- Cholesterol: 69mg
- Sodium: 747mg
- Total Carbs: 28g
- Fiber: 8g
- Sugar: 6g
- Protein: 29g
- Potassium: 1305mg

Spicy Tourne Beef

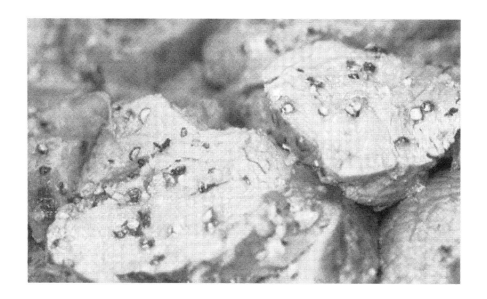

Servings: 4

Prep Time: 10 minutes

Cooking Time: 1 hour 40 minutes

Ingredients

- 3 pounds chuck roast
- 1 cup beef broth
- 1 teaspoon salt
- 1 teaspoon basil
- ¼ cup apple cider vinegar
- 1 teaspoon oregano

- 6 garlic cloves
- 1 teaspoon onion powder
- 1 teaspoon Marjoram
- ½ teaspoon ground ginger

Method

1. Take a knife and make a few incisions in the meat.
2. Press garlic cloves inside.
3. Take a small bowl and mix herbs and then rub mixture into the meat.
4. Place meat in your Instant Pot.
5. Pour vinegar and broth and lock lid.
6. Cook on HIGH pressure for 90 minutes.
7. Release pressure naturally over 10 minutes.
8. Serve and enjoy!

Nutrition information per serving

Calories: 255

Total Fat: 16g, Saturated Fat: 4g, Cholesterol: 51mg, Sodium: 351mg, Total Carbs: 8g, Fiber: 2g, Sugar: 2g, Protein: 20g, Potassium: 462mg

Balsamic Beef Delight

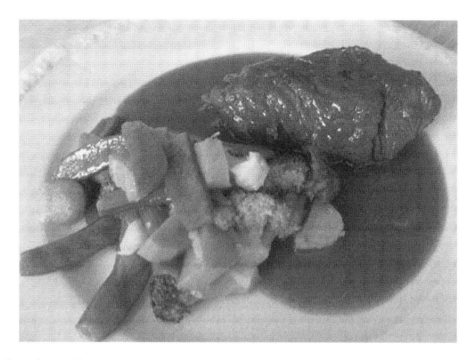

Servings: 8

Prep Time: 10 minutes

Cooking Time: 50 minutes

Ingredients

- 3 pounds chuck roast
- 3 garlic cloves, sliced
- 1 tablespoon olive oil
- 1 teaspoon flavored vinegar
- ½ teaspoon pepper
- ½ teaspoon rosemary

- 1 tablespoon clarified butter
- ½ teaspoon thyme
- ¼ cup balsamic vinegar
- 1 cup beef broth

Method

1. Cut slits in the roast and stuff with garlic slices.
2. Take a bowl and mix vinegar, rosemary, pepper, and thyme; rub all over the meat.
3. Set your pot to SAUTE mode and add roast; brown both sides (5 minutes each side).
4. Take roast out and place to the side.
5. Add butter, broth, and vinegar; deglaze the pot.
6. Transfer roast back to the pot and lock lid.
7. Cook on HIGH pressure for 40 minutes.
8. Quick release pressure.
9. Remove lid and enjoy!

Nutrition information per serving

Calories: 380

Total Fat: 23g, Saturated Fat:5g, Cholesterol: 44mg, Sodium: 448mg, Total Carbs: 24g, Fiber: 2g, Sugar: 4g, Protein: 373g, Potassium:359mg

Rich Beef Stew

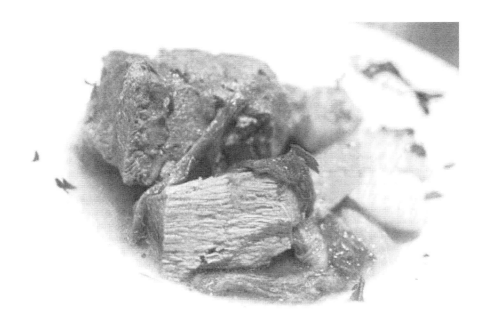

Servings: 6

Prep Time: 10 minutes

Cooking Time: 45 minutes

Ingredients

- 2 pounds beef roast, fat removed and cubed
- 4 carrots, cubed
- 2 celery stalks, chopped
- 1 yellow onion, chopped
- 2 tablespoons almond flour
- ½ cup vegetable broth

Method

1. Add beef, carrots, celery, onion, flour, and broth to the pot; stir.
2. Close lid and cook on LOW pressure for 35 minutes.
3. Release pressure naturally over 10 minutes.
4. Open the lid and divide into bowls.
5. Serve and enjoy!

Nutrition information per serving

- **Calories: 302**
- Total Fat: 8g
- Saturated Fat: 3g
- Cholesterol: 95mg
- Sodium: 698mg
- Total Carbs: 17g
- Fiber: 3g
- Sugar: 6g
- Protein: 37g
- Potassium: 1217mg

South Beef Stir Fry

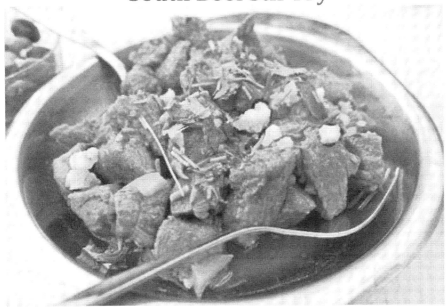

Servings: 8

Prep Time: 10 minutes

Cooking Time: 30 minutes

Ingredients

- 4 pounds beef stew meat
- 6 tablespoons coconut oil
- 4 red onions, sliced
- ½ cup ginger, chopped
- ½ cup garlic, chopped
- 1 cup coconut flakes
- 4 tablespoons fresh lemon juice

Whole Spices

- 2 teaspoons black mustard seeds
- 7 curry leaves

Spices

- 2 tablespoons meat masala
- 4 teaspoons coriander powder
- 2 teaspoons turmeric powder
- 2 teaspoons salt
- 1 teaspoon black pepper
- 1 teaspoon cayenne pepper

Method

1. Set your pot to SAUTE mode and add whole spices and coconut oil.
2. Saute for 30 seconds.
3. Add garlic, ginger, and spices.
4. Saute for 4 minutes; then add beef, lemon juice, and coconut flakes.
5. Lock lid and cook on HIGH pressure for 15 minutes.
6. Release pressure naturally over 10 minutes.
7. Stir in lemon juice.
8. Garnish with cilantro.
9. Serve and enjoy!

Nutrition information per serving

Calories: 290

Total Fat: 15g, Saturated Fat: 0g, Cholesterol: 63mg, Sodium: 607mg, Total Carbs: 15g, Fiber: 4g, Sugar: 4g, Protein: 25g, Potassium: 793mg

Original Texas Beef Chili

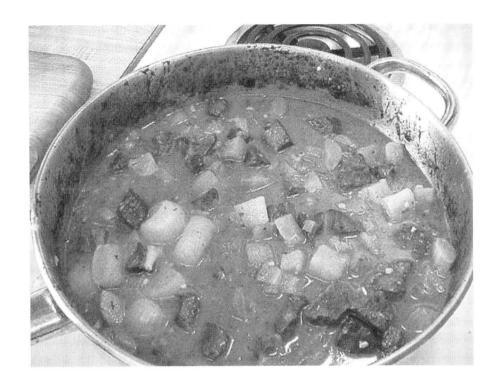

Servings: 5

Prep Time: 10 minutes

Cooking Time: 35 minutes

Ingredients

- 1 pound grass-fed organic beef
- 1 large onion, chopped
- 4 small carrots, chopped
- ½ teaspoon black pepper

- 1 teaspoon salt
- 1 teaspoon onion powder
- 1 tablespoon parsley, chopped
- 1 tablespoon Worcestershire sauce
- 4 teaspoons chili powder
- 1 teaspoon paprika
- 1 teaspoon garlic powder
- pinch of cumin

Method

1. Set your Instant Pot to "Sauté" mode, add ground beef and Saute until browned.
2. Add remaining ingredients and stir to combine.
3. Lock the lid and cook on HIGH pressure for 35 minutes on MEAT/STEW setting.
4. Release the pressure naturally over 10 minutes.
5. Open the lid and serve.
6. Enjoy!

Nutrition information per serving

Calories: 258

Total Fat: 17g, Saturated Fat: 6g, Cholesterol: 48mg, Sodium: 501mg, Total Carbs: 10g, Fiber: 2g, Sugar: 3g, Protein: 16g

Poultry Recipes

Feisty Turkey Wings

Servings: 4

Prep Time: 10 minutes

Cooking Time: 40 minutes

Ingredients

- 4 turkey wings
- 2 tablespoons clarified butter
- 2 tablespoons olive oil
- 1½ cups cranberries
- salt and pepper as needed
- 1 yellow onion, sliced
- 1 cup walnuts
- 1 cup fresh orange juice
- 1 bunch thyme, roughly chopped

Method

1. Set your pot to SAUTE mode and add butter and oil; let it heat up.
2. Add turkey wings and season with salt and pepper.
3. Brown on all sides.
4. Take wings out and place them to the side.
5. Add onions, walnuts, cranberries, and thyme; stir and cook for 2 minutes.
6. Add orange juice and then return the turkey wings to the pot.
7. Lock lid and cook on HIGH pressure for 20 minutes.
8. Release pressure naturally over 10 minutes.
9. Take the wings out and place on serving platter.
10. Set your pot to SAUTE mode and simmer the cranberry sauce for 5 minutes.
11. Drizzle sauce over wings and serve.
12. Enjoy!

Nutrition information per serving

Calories: 593

Total Fat: 27g, Saturated Fat: 27g, Cholesterol: 134mg, Sodium:485mg, Total Carbs: 43g, Fiber: 1g, Sugar: 36g, Protein: 43g, Potassium: 764mg

Amazing Chicken Primavera

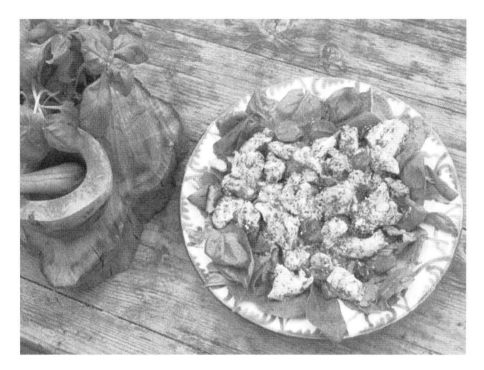

Servings: 4

Prep Time: 10 minutes

Cooking Time: 12 minutes

Ingredients

- 4 boneless chicken breasts, sliced into strips
- 1 shallot, chopped
- 6 cloves garlic, chopped
- 1 celery stalk, chopped
- 4 cups baby spinach

- ½ cup half and half
- 1 cup chicken stock
- salt and pepper to taste
- ¼ teaspoon dried mint
- ½ teaspoon dried oregano

Method

1. Add chicken breast and all remaining ingredients to your Instant Pot.
2. Stir gently to combine.
3. Lock lid and cook on HIGH pressure for 12 minutes.
4. Release the pressure naturally over 10 minutes.
5. Serve and enjoy!

Nutrition information per serving

- **Calories: 323**
- Total Fat: 14g
- Saturated Fat: 9g
- Cholesterol: 28mg
- Sodium: 312mg
- Total Carbs: 5g
- Fiber: 3g
- Sugar: 6g
- Protein: 42g
- Potassium: 551mg

Caramelized Onion Chicken

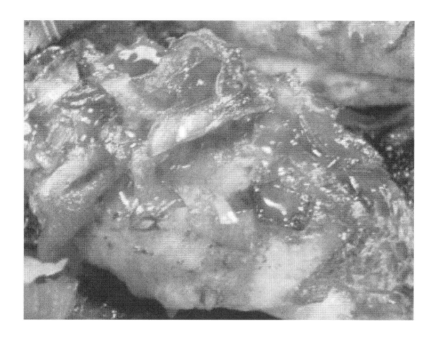

Servings: 4

Prep Time: 5 minutes

Cooking Time: 10 minutes

Ingredients

- 2 pounds boneless, skinless chicken breasts, cut into halves
- 1 teaspoon chili powder
- ½ teaspoon salt
- 1 cup lectin-free salsa
- lettuce leaves for wrapping

Method

1. Season both sides of the chicken pieces with salt.
2. Carefully arrange the chicken in a single layer in your Instant Pot.
3. Pour salsa over the chicken pieces.
4. Lock lid and cook on HIGH pressure for 7 minutes.
5. Quick release the pressure.
6. Remove lid and transfer chicken to bowl.
7. Shred the chicken using a fork and return to pot.
8. Mix to distribute shredded meat evenly throughout the sauce.
9. Serve the mixture by portioning them into individual lettuce leaf wraps.
10. Enjoy!

Nutrition information per serving

- **Calories: 407**
- Total Fat: 32g
- Saturated Fat: 4g
- Cholesterol: 46mg
- Sodium: 653mg
- Total Carbs: 13g
- Fiber: 2g
- Sugar: 20g
- Protein: 20g
- Potassium: 314mg

Simple and Precious Chinese Chicken

Servings: 4

Prep Time: 10 minutes

Cooking Time: 15 minutes

Ingredients

- 5 pounds boneless, skinless chicken thighs
- black pepper as needed
- ½ cup balsamic vinegar
- 1 teaspoon black peppercorns
- 4 cloves garlic, minced
- ½ cup coconut aminos

Method

1. Add chicken, vinegar, garlic, aminos, pepper and peppercorns to your Instant Pot.
2. Stir gently to combine.
3. Lock lid and cook on HIGH pressure for 15 minutes.
4. Release pressure naturally over 10 minutes.
5. Serve and enjoy!

Nutrition information per serving

Calories: 261

Total Fat: 7g, Saturated Fat: 2g, Cholesterol: 83mg, Sodium: 463mg,

Total Carbs: 18g, Fiber: 1g, Sugar: 3g, Protein: 8g, Potassium: 554mg

The Healthy "FAUX" Chicken Taco

Servings: 4

Prep Time: 10 minutes

Cooking Time: 15 minutes

Ingredients

- 4 chicken breasts
- 4 onions, sliced
- 2 tablespoons almond butter
- 1 tablespoon olive oil
- ½ teaspoon dried thyme
- ½ cup white wine vinegar
- 1 cup chicken stock

Method

1. Set your Instant Pot to "Sauté" mode, add almond butter and allow it to melt.
2. Add thyme, oil, and onions and saute for 10 minutes.
3. Stir in vinegar, salt, stock, pepper and carefully place the chicken on top.
4. Lock lid and cook on HIGH pressure for 10 minutes.
5. Serve and enjoy!

Nutrition information per serving

Calories: 418

Total Fat: 19g, Saturated Fat: 9g, Cholesterol: 146mg, Sodium: 1119mg, Total Carbs: 42g, Fiber: 6g, Sugar: 27g, Protein: 42g, Potassium: 1005mg

All-Time Favorite Orange Chicken

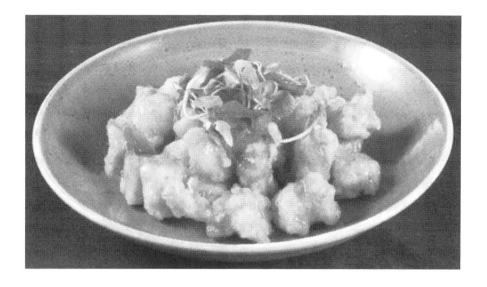

Servings: 4

Prep Time: 8 minutes

Cooking Time: 12 minutes

Ingredients

- 6 boneless, skinless chicken thighs
- 2 cloves garlic, minced
- 1 shallot, sliced
- 2 tablespoons olive oil
- 2 oranges, cut into segments
- 1 teaspoon orange zest

- 1 cup chicken stock
- salt and pepper as needed

Method

1. Set your Instant Pot to "Sauté" mode and add chicken, cook until all sides are slightly browned.
2. Cancel Saute and stir in the remaining ingredients.
3. Season with salt and pepper.
4. Lock lid and cook on HIGH pressure for 12 minutes.
5. Release pressure naturally over 10 minutes.
6. Serve and enjoy!

Nutrition information per serving

- **Calories: 337**
- Total Fat: 15g
- Saturated Fat:3g
- Cholesterol: 129mg
- Sodium: 224mg
- Total Carbs: 12g
- Fiber: 0g
- Sugar: 3g
- Protein: 41g
- Potassium: 657mg

Delicious Lemon Chicken and Cauliflower Mash

Servings: 4

Prep Time: 15 minutes

Cooking Time: 20 minutes

Ingredients

- 3 lemons, zested and juiced
- 1 teaspoon garlic powder
- 1½ teaspoons black pepper
- 2 tablespoons ghee
- 1 teaspoon salt
- 2 pounds bone-in chicken thighs
- 1 cup chicken broth
- 4 cups cauliflower, cut into large florets

Method

1. To a small bowl, add lemon zest, salt, pepper, and garlic.
2. Set your Instant Pot to "Sauté" mode and add 1 tablespoon of ghee, season the chicken thighs with lemon rub.
3. Add chicken thighs to Instant Pot and saute each side for 4 minutes.

4. Add broth to the pot and scrape any browned bits from the bottom of the pot.
5. Place trivet over chicken and layer cauliflower florets on top.
6. Season with pepper and salt.
7. Lock the lid and cook on POULTRY mode for 15 minutes.
8. Perform a quick release.
9. Open the lid and transfer cauliflower to a bowl, add 1 tablespoon of ghee and mash until desired consistency.
10. Season with salt and pepper.
11. Drizzle chicken with lemon juice.
12. Serve and enjoy!

Nutrition information per serving

- **Calories: 270**
- Total Fat: 20g
- Saturated Fat: 4g
- Cholesterol: 17mg
- Sodium: 617mg
- Total Carbs: 1g
- Fiber: 4g
- Sugar: 5g
- Protein: 20g
- Potassium: 509mg

Salad Recipes

Awesome Citrus and Cauliflower Salad

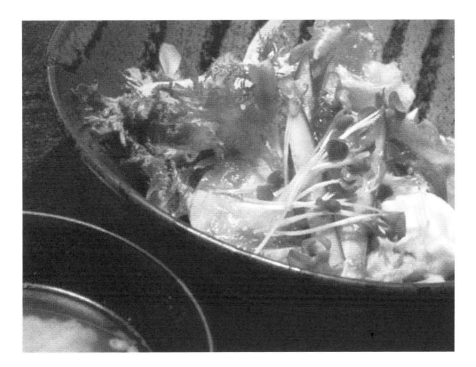

Servings: 4

Prep Time: 5 minutes

Cooking Time: 10 minutes

Ingredients

- 1 small head cauliflower, divided into florets
- 1 small Romanesco cauliflower, separated into florets
- 1 pound broccoli florets
- 2 seedless oranges, peeled and sliced

Vinaigrette

- 1 whole orange, zested and juiced
- 4 anchovies
- 1 hot pepper
- 1 tablespoon capers
- 4 tablespoons extra virgin olive oil
- salt as needed
- pepper as needed

Method

1. Add the cauliflower and broccoli to your Instant Pot.
2. Lock the lid and cook on HIGH pressure for 7 minutes.
3. Add anchovies, capers, hot pepper, pepper, olive oil, and salt to a small bowl and mix well.
4. Quick release the pressure from the Instant Pot and strain the vegetables.
5. Combine them with orange slices and vinaigrette.
6. Mix and enjoy!

Nutrition information per serving
Calories: 163

Total Fat: 11g, Saturated Fat:2g, Cholesterol: 0mg, Sodium: 488mg, Total Carbs: 8g, Fiber: 4g, Sugar: 10g, Protein: 3g, Potassium: 600mg

Extremely Hearty Beet Salad

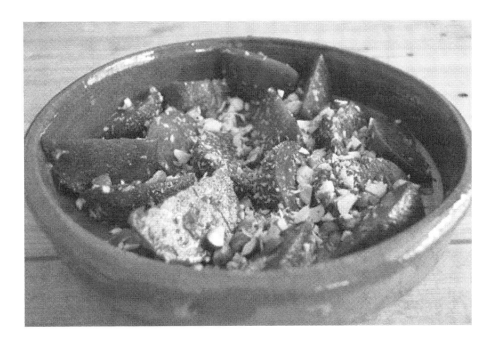

Servings: 6

Prep Time: 5 minutes

Cooking Time: 15 minutes

Ingredients

- 6 medium-sized beets
- 1 cup water
- kosher salt
- freshly ground black pepper
- balsamic vinegar
- extra virgin olive oil

Method

1. Wash the beets carefully and trim greens, leaving ½-inch of stem
2. Add 1 cup of water to the Instant Pot
3. Place steamer/trivet in a pot and arrange the beets on top of the steamer
4. Lock the lid and cook on HIGH pressure for 1 minute
5. Release the pressure naturally and allow the beets to cool
6. Carefully cut off the stem and slip the skins off the beets
7. Slice the beets into uniform pieces and season with salt and pepper
8. Add a splash of balsamic vinegar and allow them to marinate for 30 minutes
9. Drizzle with olive oil, adjust seasoning, and serve!
10. Enjoy!

Nutrition information per serving

Calories: 120

Total Fat: 7g, Saturated Fat: 3g, Cholesterol: 7mg, Sodium: 126mg, Total Carbs: 13g, Fiber: 3g, Sugar: 6g, Protein: 2g, Potassium: 304mg

Caper and Beet Salad

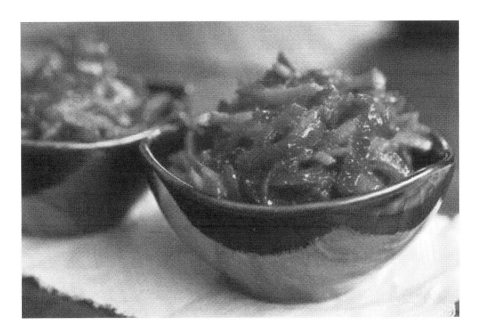

Servings: 4

Prep Time: 5 minutes

Cooking Time: 25 minutes

Ingredients

- 4 medium beets
- 2 tablespoons rice wine vinegar

For Dressing

- small bunch parsley, stems removed
- 1 large garlic clove
- ½ teaspoon salt
- pinch of black pepper

- 1 tablespoon extra virgin olive oil
- 2 tablespoons capers

Method

1. Pour 1 cup of water into your steamer basket and place it on the side.
2. Snip up the tops of your beets and wash them thoroughly.
3. Put the beets in your steamer basket.
4. Place the steamer basket in your instant pot and lock up the lid.
5. Let it cook for about 25 minutes at HIGH pressure.
6. Once done, release the pressure naturally.
7. While it is being cooked, take a small jar and add chopped up parsley and garlic alongside olive oil, salt, pepper, and capers.
8. Shake it vigorously to prepare your dressing.
9. Open up the lid once the pressure is released, and check the beets for doneness using a fork.
10. Take out the steamer basket to your sink and run it under cold water.
11. Use your finger to brush off the skin of the beets.
12. Use a plastic cutting board and slice up the beets.
13. Arrange them on a platter and sprinkle some vinegar on top.

Nutrition information per serving

Calories: 224

Total Fat: 15g, Saturated Fat: 2g, Cholesterol: 2mg, Sodium: 247mg, Total Carbs: 21g, Fiber: 6g, Sugar: 14g, Protein: 5g, Potassium: 753mg

Crazy Carrot and Kale Medley

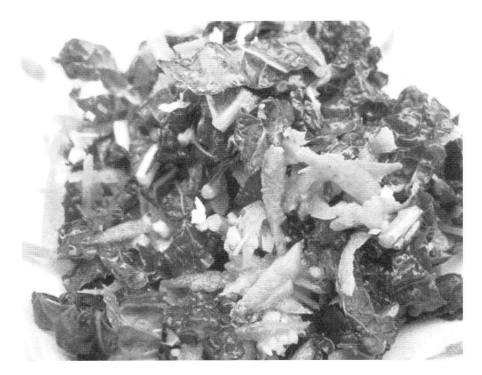

Servings: 8

Prep Time: 5 minutes

Cooking Time: 5 minutes

Ingredients

- 10 ounces kale, roughly chopped
- 1 tablespoon olive oil
- 1 medium onion, thinly sliced
- 3 medium carrots, cut into ½-inch slices
- 5 cloves garlic, chopped
- ½ cup chicken broth

- kosher salt as needed
- freshly ground pepper
- aged balsamic vinegar
- ¼ teaspoon red pepper flakes

Method

1. Set your Instant Pot to "Sauté" mode and add olive oil, let the oil heat up.
2. Add chopped carrots and onions, saute for a few minutes.
3. Add garlic and stir for 30 seconds.
4. Add kale and vegetable broth.
5. Season with salt and pepper.
6. Lock lid and cook on HIGH pressure for 5 minutes.
7. Release pressure over 10 minutes.
8. Stir well.
9. Season with salt and pepper.
10. Drizzle with balsamic vinegar and sprinkle red pepper flakes over the top.
11. Serve and enjoy!

Nutrition information per serving

Calories: 232

Total Fat: 14g, Saturated Fat: 0g, Cholesterol: 0mg, Sodium: 257mg, Total Carbs: 21g, Fiber: 11g, Sugar: 3g, Protein: 10g, Potassium:1212mg

Desserts Recipes

Cool Peppermint Latte

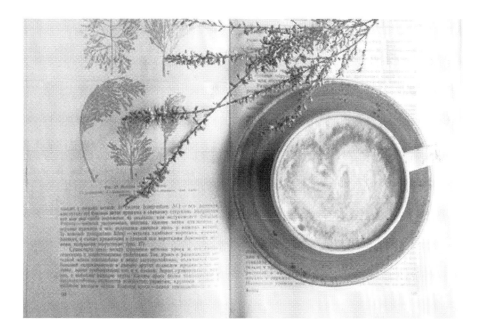

Servings: 4

Prep Time: 5 minutes

Cooking Time: 5 minutes

Ingredients

- 4 cups almond milk
- 2 cups coffee
- 1 teaspoon vanilla bean extract
- 23 drops peppermint oil

Method

1. Add all of the listed ingredients to your pot.
2. Lock up the lid and cook on HIGH pressure for 5 minutes.
3. Allow the pot to release pressure naturally.
4. Open the pot and serve!

Nutrition information per serving

- Calories: 169
- Total Fat: 9g
- Saturated Fat: 6g
- Cholesterol: 28mg
- Sodium: 68mg
- Total Carbs: 14g
- Fiber: 0g
- Sugar: 12g
- Protein: 4g
- Potassium: 297mg

Very Creamy Mashed Sweet Potatoes

Servings: 2

Prep Time: 5 minutes

Cooking Time: 20 minutes

Ingredients

- 2 pounds garnet sweet potatoes, cut into 1-inch chunks
- 2-3 tablespoons clarified butter
- 2 tablespoons stevia
- ¼ teaspoon nutmeg
- 1 cup water
- salt as needed

Method

1. Peel the sweet potatoes and cut up into 1-inch chunks.
2. Pour 1 cup of water to the pot and add steamer basket.
3. Add sweet potato chunks in the basket.
4. Lock up the lid and cook on HIGH pressure for 8 minutes.
5. Quick release the pressure.
6. Open the lid and place the cooked sweet potatoes in the bowl.
7. Use a masher to mash the potatoes.

8. Add ¼ teaspoon of nutmeg, 2-3 tablespoon of clarified butter, 2 tablespoons of stevia.
9. Mash and mix.
10. Season with salt.
11. Serve and enjoy!

Nutrition information per serving

- **Calories: 115**
- Total Fat: 1g
- Saturated Fat: 0g
- Cholesterol: 1mg
- Sodium: 1mg
- Total Carbs: 24g
- Fiber: 3g
- Sugar: 5g
- Protein: 4g
- Potassium: 232mg

Peachy Raspberry Lemonade

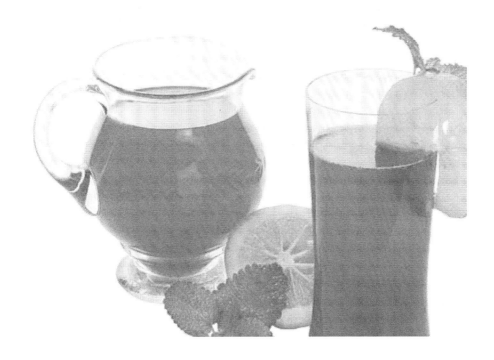

Servings: 4

Prep Time: 5 minutes

Cooking Time: 5 minutes

Ingredients

- 1 cup peaches, chopped
- ½ cup raspberries
- zest and juice of 1 lemon

Method

1. Add listed ingredients to your Instant Pot.
2. Add a cup of water (more if needed, the objective is to barely cover the contents).
3. Lock lid and cook on HIGH pressure for 5 minutes.
4. Quick release pressure.
5. Drain the juice.
6. Serve the juice chilled and enjoy!

Nutrition information per serving

- **Calories: 111**
- Total Fat: 0g
- Saturated Fat: 0g
- Cholesterol: 0mg
- Sodium: 6mg
- Total Carbs: 3g
- Fiber: 0g
- Sugar: 3g
- Protein: 0g
- Potassium: 9mg

Hearty Coconut and Avocado Pudding

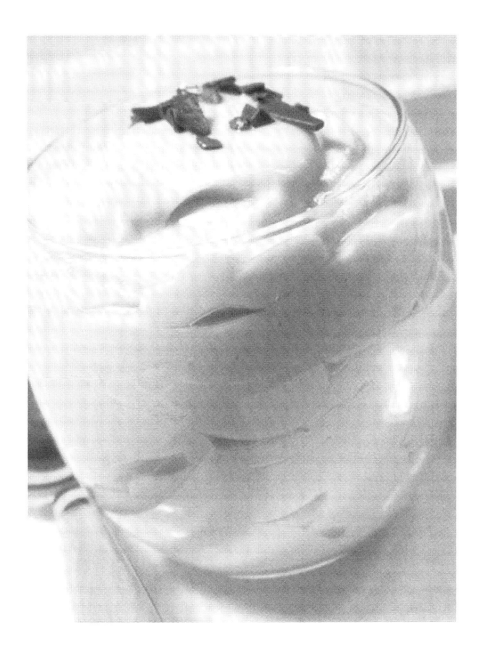

Servings: 4

Prep Time: 10 minutes

Cooking Time: 15 minutes

Ingredients

- 2 avocados, pitted, peeled and chopped
- 2 teaspoons vanilla bean extract
- 2 tablespoons coconut sugar
- 1 tablespoon lime juice
- 1 can (14.5 ounces) coconut milk
- 1½ cups water

Method

1. Take a bowl and add coconut milk, vanilla bean extract, avocado, coconut sugar, and lime juice; blend.
2. Pour mix into a ramekin.
3. Add water to your Instant Pot.
4. Place a steamer basket in your Instant Pot.
5. Add ramekin to the basket.
6. Lock lid and cook on HIGH pressure for 5 minutes.
7. Release pressure naturally over 10 minutes.
8. Serve and enjoy!

Nutrition information per serving

Calories: 432

Total Fat: 20g, Saturated Fat: 5g, Cholesterol: 0mg, Sodium: 41mg, Total Carbs: 74g, Fiber: 17g, Sugar: 20g, Protein: 6g, Potassium: 41mg

Easy Baked Apple

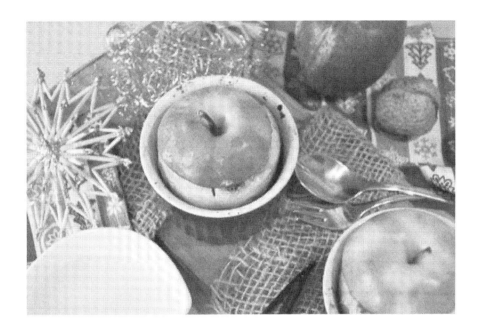

Servings: 5

Prep Time: 5 minutes

Cooking Time: 5 minutes

Ingredients

- 6 fresh apples, cored, peeled, and sliced
- ¼ cup raisins
- 1 cup red wine vinegar
- 1 teaspoon cinnamon powder

Method

1. Add apples to your Instant Pot.
2. Add vinegar, cinnamon, and raisins, and stir.
3. Lock lid and cook on HIGH pressure for 10 minutes.
4. Release the pressure naturally over 10 minutes.
5. Scoop into bowls and serve with a drizzle of cooking liquid on top.
6. Enjoy!

Nutrition information per serving

- **Calories: 332**
- Total Fat: 17g
- Saturated Fat: 5
- Cholesterol: 34mg
- Sodium: 145mg
- Total Carbs: 45g
- Fiber: 3g
- Sugar: 34g
- Protein: 3g
- Potassium: 7g

Creative Stinking Rose

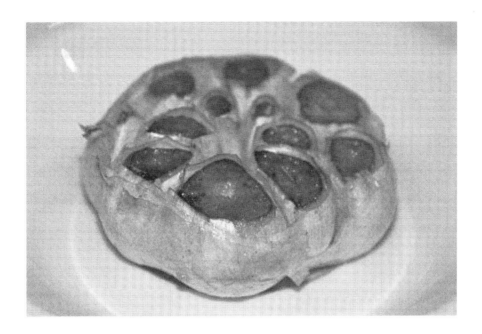

Servings: 4

Prep Time: 5 minutes

Cooking Time: 55 minutes

Ingredients

- 3 large garlic bulbs, whole
- drizzle of extra virgin olive oil
- 1 cup water

Method

1. Place steamer rack inside your Instant Pot.
2. Add water.
3. Trim off top ¼-inch of garlic bulb Transfer the garlic bulbs to the steamer rack.
4. Lock lid and cook on HIGH pressure for 6 minutes.
5. Release pressure naturally over 10 minutes.
6. Remove garlic using tongs and transfer to an oven-safe dish.
7. Drizzle oil over garlic bulbs and broil for 55 minutes.
8. Serve and enjoy!

Nutrition information per serving

- **Calories: 254**
- Total Fat: 16g
- Saturated Fat: 1g
- Cholesterol: 0mg
- Sodium: 220mg
- Total Carbs: 19g
- Fiber: 2g
- Sugar: 1g
- Protein: 9g
- Potassium: 350mg

Hearty Sweet and Spicy Carrot

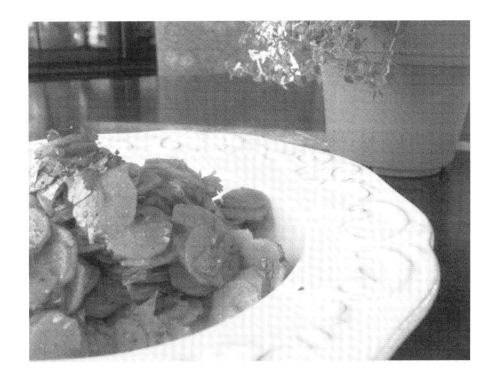

Servings: 4

Prep Time: 5 minutes

Cooking Time: 2 minutes

Ingredients

- 1 cup water
- 5-6 large carrots, peeled and cut into 1-inch chunks
- 1 tablespoon clarified butter
- ¼ teaspoon ground cumin

- ¼ teaspoon cayenne
- salt and pepper
- 2 teaspoons honey

Method

1. Add water to your Instant Pot.
2. Insert steamer basket.
3. Add carrots.
4. Lock lid and STEAM for 2 minutes on high pressure.
5. Quick release pressure.
6. Remove steamer basket and pour the water out.
7. Dry the pot and place it in the Instant Pot again.
8. Add clarified butter to the pot and set it to Saute mode.
9. Add carrots to the pot and stir until coated with butter.
10. Add cumin and cayenne and season with salt and pepper.
11. Stir well.
12. Add honey and Cancel Saute.
13. Stir.
14. Serve and enjoy!

Nutrition information per serving

Calories: 74

Total Fat: 4g, Saturated Fat: 2g, Cholesterol: 0mg, Sodium: 122mg, Total Carbs: 20g, Fiber: 2g, Sugar: 11g, Protein: 1g, Potassium: 549mg

Cooking Measurement Conversion

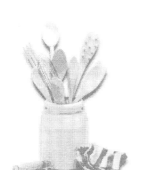

US Dry Volume Measurements

1/16 teaspoon	a dash
1/8 teaspoon	a pinch
3 teaspoons	1 tablespoon
¼ cup	4 tablespoons
1/3 cup	5 tablespoons + 1 teaspoon
½ cup	8 tablespoons
¾ cup	12 tablespoons
1 cup	16 tablespoons
1 pound	16 ounces

US Liquid Volume Measurements

8 fluid ounces	1 cup
1 pint = 2 cups	16 fluid ounces
1 quart = 2 pints	4 cups
1 gallon = 4 quarts	16 cups

Grocery Shopping List

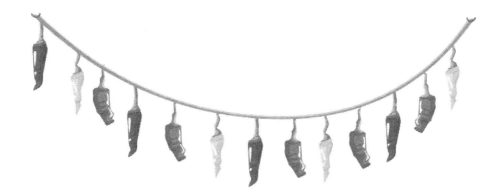

Flours
- [ ] Almond Flour

Dairy
- [ ] Coconut Milk
- [ ] Almond Milk
- [ ] Almond Butter
- [ ] Ghee

Seafood
- [ ] Tilapia
- [ ] Salmon
- [ ] Crab
- [ ] Sea Bass
- [ ] Anchovies

Nuts and Seeds
- [ ] Almond
- [ ] Mustard Seeds
- [ ] Sesame Seeds
- [ ] Coconut Flakes
- [ ] Walnut
- [ ] Cashews

Meat
- [ ] Chicken
- [ ] Chuck Roast
- [ ] Bacon
- [ ] Beef
- [ ] Pork
- [ ] Turkey Wings

Oils, Vinegar, & Condiments

- Extra-virgin Olive Oil
- Sesame Oil
- Coconut Oil
- Peppermint Oil
- Fish Sauce
- Sriracha Sauce
- Worcestershire Sauce
- Vinegar
- Balsamic Glaze
- Capers

Vegetables

- Bella Mushrooms
- Onion
- Carrots
- Beet
- Cabbage
- Kale
- Cauliflower
- Broccoli
- Brussels Sprouts
- Sweet Potato
- Leek
- Celery
- Chard
- Pumpkin
- Bok Choy
- Parsnip
- Artichoke

Dried Herbs, Vegetables & Spices

- Oregano
- Rosemary
- Garlic Powder
- Thyme
- Coconut aminos
- Marjoram
- Coriander
- Mint
- Chili

Seasonings

- Salt
- Coconut Sugar
- Vanilla Bean Extract
- Stevia
- Cinnamon
- Pepper
- Spinach
- Garlic
- Ginger
- Chive
- Sage
- Letucce
- Scallion
- Basil
- Bay Leaf
- Thyme
- Lemon
- Parsley
- Cilantro

Fruits

- [ ] Apple
- [ ] Orange
- [ ] Pineapple
- [ ] Lime
- [ ] Cranberry
- [ ] Raspberry
- [ ] Avocado

- [ ] Nutmeg
- [ ] Cumin
- [ ] Paprika
- [ ] Masala
- [ ] Curry
- [ ] Turmeric

Beverages

- [ ] Chicken Broth
- [ ] Vegetable Broth
- [ ] Beef Broth
- [ ] Coffee

Sweets

- [ ] Raisings
- [ ] Coconut Cream
- [ ] Date Paste

Our recommendations

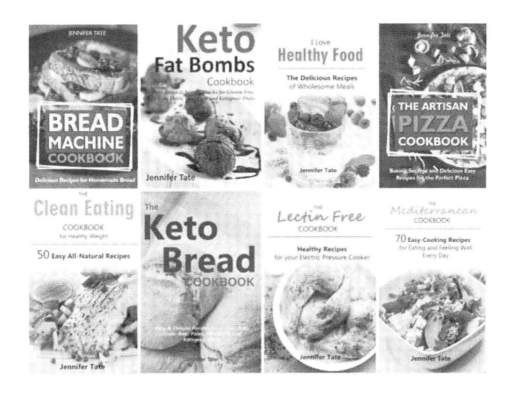

About the Author

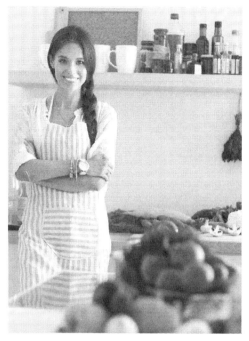

I am a **professional nutritionist**. I have been researching various diets and their effects on human health for 15 years already.

Sometimes only with the help of specialized nutrition, you can improve a person's condition without resorting to medication.

I liked the lectin-free diet right away. **It can reduce inflammation in the body, help you to lose weight and prevent many diseases.**

I will not say that it is easy to follow. But in this book, I have collected the recipes for you that will help you get rid of diseases and enjoy your life without stress.

My clients are delighted with the results of the lectin-free diet, and from time to time they apply it to **solve their health problems.** It can also be used to **maintain your weight.**

The Lectin Free Cookbook is made with love and experienced.

Recipe Index

A

Advantages of Instant Pot 18
All-Time Favorite Orange Chicken 99
Amazing Chicken Primavera 93
Awesome Citrus and Cauliflower Salad 103
Awesome Parsnips and Chive Soup 35

B

Balsamic Beef Delight 83

BASICS OF THE LECTIN FREE DIET 9

BEEF RECIPES 77

Benefits of a Lectin Free Diet 13
Broccoli and Ginger Beef 79

C

Caper and Beet Salad 107
Caramelized Onion Chicken 95
Chicken Kale Soup 20
Chicken Turmeric Soup 22

COOKING MEASUREMENT CONVERSION 125

Cool Instant Pot Broccoli 33
Cool Peppermint Latte 111
Crazy Carrot and Kale Medley 109

Creamy Leek and Broccoli Soup 45
Creative Stinking Rose 121

D

Delicious Bowl of Mushrooms 39
Delicious Lemon Chicken and Cauliflower Mash 101

DESSERTS RECIPES 111

E

Easy Baked Apple 119
Easy Jamaican Pork 68
Exotic Chili and Garlic Beef 77
Extremely Hearty Beet Salad 105

F

Fantastic Ginger Tilapia 51
Feisty Pot of Brussels Sprouts 43
Feisty Turkey Wings 91

G

Garlic and Broccoli Mash 47
Gentle Crab Legs 56

H

Hamburger Vegetable Soup 29

Healthy Carrot Soup 49

Hearty Coconut and Avocado Pudding 117

Hearty Lemon and Artichoke Pork Chops 62

Hearty Sweet and Spicy Carrot 123

How Lectins Can Harm Your Health? 10

I

Juicy Coconut Fish Curry 60

L

Lectin-Free Pantry Staples and Seasonings 14

O

Olive Dredged Pork Belly 75

Onion Pork Bliss 66

Original Texas Beef Chili 89

P

Peachy Raspberry Lemonade 115

Pepper Lemon Salmon 54

PORK RECIPES 62

POULTRY RECIPES 91

R

Rich Beef Stew 85

Roasted Garlic Soup 27

S

SALAD RECIPES 103

SEAFOOD RECIPES 51

Sesame Bok Choy Platter 31

Shredded Cabbage and Bacon 72

Simple and Precious Chinese Chicken 97

Slightly Spicy Chili Salmon 58

SOUPS 20

South Beef Stir Fry 87

Spicy Tourne Beef 81

Sprouts and Chops Medley 70

Subtle Braised Cabbage 37

T

Tender Soft Pineapple Pork Chops 64

Thai Broccoli and Beef Soup 25

The "Ghee"- Licious Pork Chops 73

The Healthy "FAUX" Chicken Taco 98

V

VEGETABLE RECIPES 31

    Very Creamy Mashed Sweet Potatoes 113

W

    What are Lectins? 9
    What is a Lectin Free Diet? 11
    What is an Instant Pot? 17

Y

    Yummy Roasted Artichoke Platter 41

Copyright

ALL ©COPYRIGHTS RESERVED 2018 by Jennifer Tate

All Rights Reserved. *No part of this publication or the information in it may be quoted from or reproduced in any form by means such as printing, scanning, photocopying or otherwise without prior written permission of the copyright holder.*

Disclaimer and Terms of Use*: Effort has been made to ensure that the information in this book is accurate and complete; however, the author and the publisher do not warrant the accuracy of the information, text, or graphics contained within the book due to the rapidly changing nature of science, research, known and unknown facts, and the internet. The author and the publisher do not hold any responsibility for errors, omissions, or contrary interpretation of the subject matter herein. This book is presented solely for motivational and informational purposes only.*

Made in the USA
San Bernardino, CA
10 April 2019